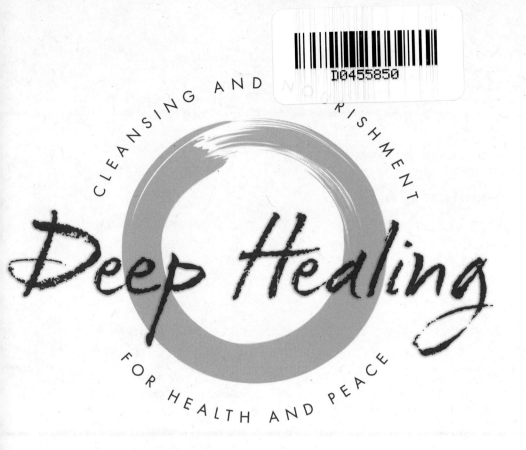

Deep Healing

CLEANSING AND NOURISHMENT

FOR HEALTH AND PEACE

Caroline Marie Dupont

books Alive

Summertown
TENNESSEE

Library of Congress Cataloging-in-Publication Data

Dupont, Caroline Marie.
    Deep healing : cleansing and nourishment for health and peace / Caroline Marie
Dupont.
        pages cm
    Includes index.
    ISBN 978-0-920470-85-5 (pbk.)
    1. Detoxification (Health)   2. Spiritual healing.   3. Reducing diets—Recipes.
I. Title.
    RA1213.D87 2014
    613.2—dc23

                                                                    2013043687

Book Publishing Company is a member of Green Press Initiative. We chose to print this title on paper with 100% postconsumer recycled content, processed without chlorine, which saves the following natural resources:

- 35 trees
- 1,103 pounds of solid waste
- 16, 846 gallons of water
- 3,040 pounds of greenhouse gases
- 16 million BTU of energy

For more information on Green Press Initiative, visit greenpressinitiative.org.

 green press INITIATIVE

Printed on recycled paper

Environmental impact estimates were made using the Environmental Defense Fund Paper Calculator. For more information, visit papercalculator.org.

Cover photo: Celine Saki
Cover and interior design: John Wincek
Stock photography: 123 RF

Printed in Canada

ISBN 13: 978-0-92047-085-5

Published by Books Alive, an imprint of
Book Publishing Company
P.O. Box 99
Summertown, TN 38483
888-260-8458
bookpubco.com

19 18 17 16 15 14   1 2 3 4 5 6 7 8 9

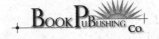

To body.

To soul.

To Life.

To you.

Contents

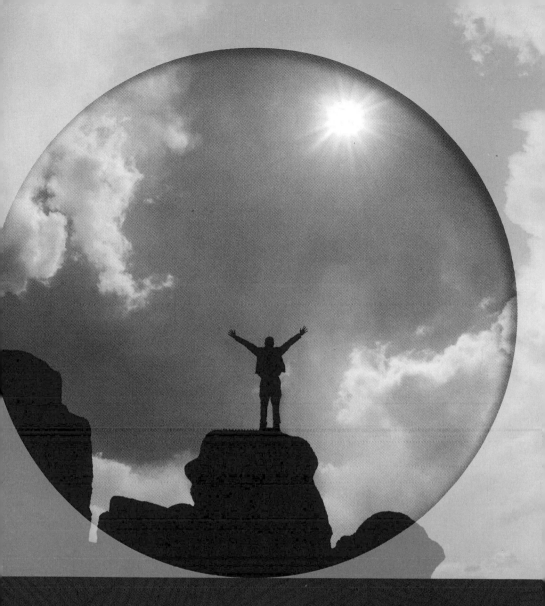

Preface

"And I saw a new Heaven and a new Earth . . .
I heard a voice saying there shall be no more death,
neither sorrow, nor crying, for the former things have passed away."

ESSENE BOOK OF REVELATIONS,
TRANSLATED BY EDMOND BORDEAUX SZEKELY

*M*y personal experience with deep healing and my many years as a holistic health practitioner and teacher have demonstrated unequivocally that an integrated approach to health is the only way to get at the root cause of disease. That's why I incorporate a variety of vital techniques into my healing practices including meditation, juice fasting, cleansing, and a wholesome plant-based diet. In this book, I share the deep insights I've gained through my life and work so that you too can learn and use them to prevent or overcome any health concerns you may have.

Although I've never developed a serious disease, I believe that if I had not begun to incorporate the principles and practices that I share in this book I would have eventually. My own health and spiritual awakening began in earnest in my late twenties, around the time that my children were born. Previously, particularly in my teens and early adulthood, I was pretty asleep to who I really was. I was shy, insecure, guarded, and often irritated and judgmental. After I had my children, I was exposed to many new things that inspired me: vegetarian diet, holistic nutrition, intuitive movement, energy work, yoga, meditation, and many things that had not previously been in my life. In many ways, it was exhilarating. At the same time, I became painfully aware of the emotions that I had been carrying and of the unhealthy patterns that ran through many aspects of my life. The next ten years were extremely challenging. They included my marriage ending, financial struggles, losing my home, and challenges in my role as a mother.

I remember waking up one night with a persistent pain in my lower abdomen, with a sudden and deep knowing that it was time to take an honest look at my life or I would get sick.

However, in my early forties—despite trying to eat right, exercise, meditate, and take care of my emotional life—health challenges started surfacing. I found myself waking up in the middle of the night, unable to go back to sleep. I had low energy, poor digestion, gum disease, and restless legs syndrome, and, most frightening of all, a Pap smear revealed abnormal cells on my cervix. Although I've had an inherent trust in the body's ability to heal itself as long as I can remember, these issues were clearly a sign that I needed to open to deeper approaches to the healing process.

I visited a local naturopath and, after some tests, she told me my body had high toxicity levels and I was at risk for cancer. I immediately told myself that her machines were faulty, but clearly a part of me knew it was true because I broke down and cried in the car on the way home. How could this be? I thought I took excellent care of myself; I ate a vegetarian diet and made most of my food from scratch. I purchased organic food and didn't drink alcohol. I exercised and meditated regularly. As a nutritionist, energy worker, and yoga and meditation teacher, I was even teaching others how to be healthy! I felt discouraged, angry, scared, and confused.

I began to focus more on my body during my meditations and started receiving information and guidance. During one sitting, I was meditating on my liver, and a memory from my childhood suddenly came back to me with great clarity and detail. My sister and I were staining a fence and decided to paint our entire bodies with the solvent my mom had given us to clean the brushes. During my meditation, I could clearly see that my liver had gone into "shock" as a result of that incident and that it was still feeling the energetic and chemical effects decades later. I went to see another naturopath who confirmed the toxic state of my liver and the presence of solvents in my body.

In order to heal my cervix, I realized I had to address the toxic burden my body was carrying. Since the liver is the primary organ of detoxification, it needed to be my focus. From the energy work I had practiced, I was aware that the liver also holds anger. In order to heal, I needed to find a way to let go of the tension of anger and other repressed emotions, so that life force and nourishment could flow in and suppressed energies and toxins could flow out.

Over the course of the next several months, I completely dedicated myself to my healing. Of particular importance was sitting in silence every day and trusting my body to guide me to the lifestyle choices that were needed. It wasn't always clear, and there were often challenges, but in retrospect I realize that I was receiving intuitive guidance all along the way. I shifted my diet to include more living foods, eliminated dairy products, and stopped using heated oils. I went on a juice fast, received energy work from a friend, attended counseling sessions, and committed to going to bed early most nights. I also attended a few silent retreats. These were particularly instrumental because they enabled me to relax into an ever-deepening spiritual stability. From this I could bring greater awareness to the whole complex of conditioning that had led to the many suppressed emotions and blocked energies that I was carrying.

Later that year I returned to my naturopath to be tested. To her surprise, and my delight, all of my physical issues had either stopped progressing or had reversed. Today, I feel content and well in my body. I do my best to honor and value it for the gift that it is. Although it's not always easy, I continue to see my emotions as beautiful teachers. My greatest longing is to know and express who I truly am, and awakening is my priority. Every moment, challenging or easy, is a precious moment. I am touched by the beauty of Life as it is and am often awed by the perfection I sense in every moment. My heart-felt hope is that the guidance presented in this book will contribute to the unveiling of all that you are.

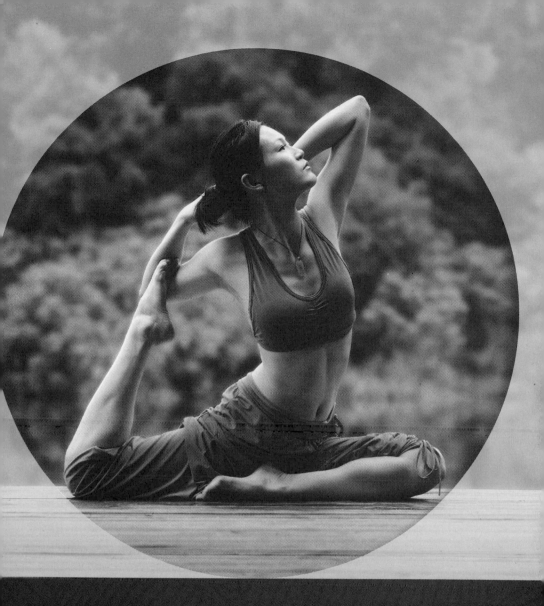

Introduction

"Honor your body, which is your representative in this universe.
Its magnificence is no accident. It is the framework through which your works
must come; through which the spirit and the spirit within the spirit speaks.
The flesh and the spirit are two phases of your actuality in space and time.
Who ignores one, falls apart in shambles. So it is written."

THE SACRED SCRIPT OF THE COVENANT (AN ANCIENT SUMARI TEXT)

*A*s a holistic health practitioner, nutritionist, and energy worker, I have seen all around me the undeniable evidence that our bodies, with the help of our minds and souls, have the ability to reverse disease so we can thrive and live vibrantly. Yes, that's right: you can heal yourself. And you can *heal deeply* if you take responsibility for your emotional well-being and spiritual growth as well as your physical health. If you're willing to surrender to the wisdom of your body and soul, this book is the perfect guide to show you how. And that can mean not only recovering from illness but preventing it as well.

Humans are spiritual beings living in physical bodies, so we experience the joy of the soul expressing itself in physical form. But the reverse can also be true: we can become ill when the soul longs for but is denied fulfillment. I believe the strongest force in the universe is the soul's desire to reveal its true nature, and physical symptoms and conditions often let us know when the soul is suffering or, in other words, when we're not being our authentic selves. When you fully express your true nature, your actions benefit not only you but also your family, community, and all life on earth.

While your health is your responsibility, it's certainly not your fault if your true nature has been stifled or if you become ill, and you're surely not alone. Many sincere people flounder in their efforts to heal; in part, this is caused by conditioning. When we're young, parents, teachers, and others who are influential in our lives may be more inclined to mold us in a manner that serves their own needs (or conditioning) rather than our needs.

From our earliest days, we're programmed to respond to external motivation rather than follow our innate wisdom and strive for authentic expression. Naturally, we become conflicted over time. We get stuck in false beliefs and our emotional energy stagnates. To heal deeply, we must be willing to challenge false beliefs, even though doing so feels uncomfortable. Another painful but essential process is releasing blocked emotional energy, which is the root cause of disease and poor lifestyle choices. Despite our good intentions, all too often we fall into habits that may temporarily satisfy us but erode our health over the long term.

Conditioning, false beliefs, and blocked emotional energy are not the only barriers to deep healing. Many other influences—including big business, culture, industrialization, media, modern medicine, organized religion, and science—can contribute to a disdain for and mistrust of the body and alienate us from our essential spiritual nature. The body, mind, and emotions need to work together in deep healing, and that's why it's so important to learn to listen to ourselves. Think of this inside voice as your intuition or your soul, an able teacher on your healing journey, and trust and rely on it.

There's never been a better time to explore the rewards of deep healing. In this powerful age of unsurpassed human physical and spiritual evolution, there are spiritual practices and lifestyle choices that make a difference. For example, awareness and intuition are aided by meditation and an understanding of how energy works in ourselves and in the universe. These topics are covered in chapters 2, 3, and 4 and can help you find and express your true nature over time.

Another aspect of deep healing is effectively learning how to eliminate toxins, which can come from many sources and affect us not only physically but also mentally and emotionally. Chapter 5 explores elimination and detoxification.

One of the most effective tools we can use when we seek deep healing is the juice fast. Particularly when used in conjunction with other cleansing practices, the juice fast can accentuate and accelerate your physical and spiritual evolution. Chapter 6 highlights the juice fast, and chapter 7 explores other cleansing practices that can promote well-being.

Another cornerstone of deep healing is a wholesome diet. Regrettably, as a society and as individuals, we've gone very far astray in our food choices in this modern age. We've forgotten what a tremendous impact food has on our bodies, our mental and emotional states, and our ability to make spiritual connections. Our healing increases dramatically when we adopt a whole-foods, plant-based diet and make choices that promote harmony with our natural surroundings. In a broader sense, our food choices greatly affect our capacity to live authentically and to heal when we recognize our profound interdependence with each other, the animals, the plants, and other beings. Chapter 8 examines the deep-healing diet, which encourages the consumption of living foods. A small collection of recipes (see pages 85 to 119) will introduce you to nourishing beverages, from tea infusions to mineral broths to smoothies and fresh juices, and endlessly versatile main dishes, such as the Hearty Salad Meal and Heaven on Earth Bowl.

You'll likely find statements in this book that resonate with you immediately; in effect, you'll be reading what your soul already knows. At other times, the content of this book may challenge your long-held beliefs. When that happens, observe what you're feeling. My hope is that as you assimilate the following information with your own innate healing wisdom, you'll come to better understand the process of deep healing. Relax into it. Feel the magic and mystery of it. Most important, see your healing as a journey back to the perfection of who and what you've always been. Then get on with being the most vital and most evolved version of yourself. Let's get started.

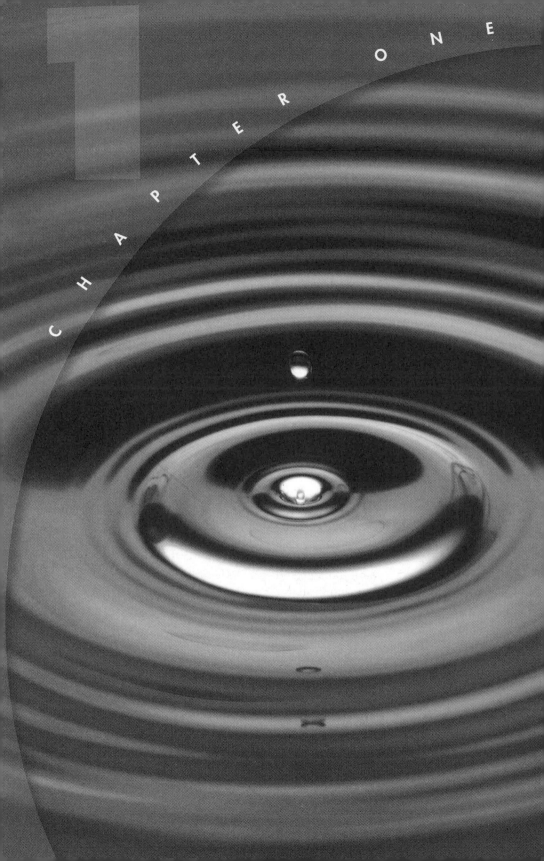

CHAPTER ONE

Deep Healing Basics

May you be well in body and mind. May you be peaceful
and truly happy. May you be filled with loving-kindness.
May you enjoy the gifts of your talents and abilities. May
you accept what is.

ADAPTATION OF THE BUDDHIST METTA PRACTICE

The root of the English word "heal" is derived from the Anglo-Saxon word
haelen, which means to be or become whole. This notion of becoming, or
transforming, is important because it emphasizes that healing is a process,
not an end point. It means we work toward being whole in each moment, one
moment at a time, and not at some point in the future. To be whole then, is to
accept what is and to be balanced in body, mind, and spirit.

The journey toward wholeness begins and is sustained when we adopt healing
behaviors and tend to ourselves with loving attention. Just as a successful gardener knows that plants need certain essentials to thrive, we understand innately that
there's a similar formula that can help us achieve all that is possible for ourselves—
physically, mentally, and spiritually.

A FORMULA FOR DEEP HEALING

In general, our physical, mental, and spiritual needs overlap because we
can't neatly separate the soul from the body, or even from the mind, for
that matter. They profoundly affect each other because they're all made
of the same fabric, which is energy. One essential aspect of a deep-healing practice is becoming aware of our own energy patterns. For example, does our energy
flow freely or is it blocked by negative emotions? Meditation is a particularly
valuable deep-healing practice that aids in energy awareness, helps us become
our authentic selves, and teaches us to tap into our own healing intuition.

DEEP HEALING
An Opportunity

Deep healing is an invitation to seeing and accepting the world as it is. In addition, deep healing is an opportunity to reflect on what you really want from life. What is your deepest aspiration? Uncover it and work toward it every day. Make it the criteria for every action and word.

Through healing, you're not required to create a new you. In fact, the opposite is true. Healing is about recovering your authenticity. It is about accessing the truth and beauty that have always been a part of you. The more deeply you connect with your true self, the more intuitive guidance you will receive. All aspects of your life will heal in accordance with your unique contract and purpose.

The physical habits that support deep healing include nutrition and cleansing (or detoxification). I recommend a plant-based diet with a focus on living foods (also called raw foods) and whole foods. In addition, I recommend periodic juice fasts in conjunction with ongoing cleansing practices, and these concepts are explored in detail in the following chapters. Here is a summary of the topics we'll explore together in the pages that follow:

Energy Awareness

Energy awareness means tuning in to the energy sensations in our bodies. When emotional energy is stuck, our bodies are literally operating at lower frequencies and therefore subject to physical illness. When energy, which is sometimes called chi or prana, is flowing, deep healing is possible. One practice that can improve energy flow and put us in a more positive state is meditation.

Meditation and Spiritual Healing

Meditation, in one form or another, is a core practice in all spiritual traditions. The deep-healing meditation included in this book provides a step-by-step method for bringing awareness to what's happening to you on a physical, mental, and emotional level. In the simplest terms, meditation is one method that can help you learn to listen to yourself to support deep healing. For more information, see "Deep Listening: Observe and Heal," page 3.

Cleansing

When excess toxins accumulate in the body, they can contribute to disease, not to mention mental and emotional imbalance. Cleansing practices help to remove these toxins. The juice fast is a very powerful cleansing tool because it provides valuable nutrients in liquid form, giving the body

Observe and Heal

You're the expert on you. Nobody knows you as well as you do—and nobody knows what you need to heal better than you. Learning to listen to yourself is one of the keys to healing. What does your intuition tell you? What messages are you getting in your dreams, during meditation, or as you go about your daily activities? Why is a particular memory significant for you at this time? How does your body feel at certain times, such as after you've eaten? Throughout this book, look for suggestions on how to listen deeply. Take heed: what are you trying to tell yourself?

a chance to work less diligently on digestion and focus on eliminating built-up toxins. Various other cleansing practices can be used to augment a fast or can be incorporated into your daily regimen.

The Everyday Deep-Healing Diet

Deep healing is aided by a plant-based diet consisting of many whole foods like fruits, vegetables, grains, legumes, and nuts. Whenever feasible, buy locally grown organic produce or grow your own. Animal-based foods are well-known contributors to most deadly diseases, including cancer, heart disease, and diabetes. Most are also produced on massive, industrialized "farms," where animals are denied the opportunity to live according to their natural instincts. That's why meat, dairy, and egg products not only contain harmful antibiotics, bacteria, and growth hormones but also transmit the energy of miserable and terrified animals.

CHOICES

As a holistic health practitioner, I seek to have a balanced, fulfilled, healthy, and joyful life, and my dharma is to guide others to do the same. The good and bad news is that I have ample opportunity: all around me I see people struggling to find balance in their lives, and I see the physical and emotional suffering that results. I live with this question: why don't people consistently take care of themselves (body and soul) when it clearly creates the foundation for the true happiness they deeply want?

It seems to me there's an abundant amount of information on how to take care of the body and soul today. And yet I often hear clients, friends, and students say they can't find the energy, motivation, or time to make food from scratch, meditate, go for walks, go to bed early, and otherwise take care of themselves. They say they know they should do these things and that they feel more balanced and connected when they do, but somehow life gets in the way.

We are all creating our lives on a moment-to-moment basis and our choices depend on what we are valuing most at any given time.

Internal and External Values

Many of us are driven by external and conditioned values, such as accomplishing goals, building wealth, conforming to rigid definitions of beauty, getting things done, pleasing others, receiving public recognition, and seeking immediate comfort or pleasure. Basing our choices on external values, however, prevents us from discovering and being our authentic selves and may interfere with our ability to heal.

So how do we shift from making choices based on external values to relying instead on internal ones? My experience is that life will often force us to, one way or the other. Our priorities shift when we suffer setbacks in life, such as when our health is failing or we're struggling financially. A change can also be triggered when we no longer have the energy to drive ourselves to achieve or push ourselves to check off tasks on a to-do list. Or we turn to our internal values when we realize that any kind of addiction or desire for immediate pleasure costs us more than it gives us, or when the people around us disapprove of us or seem unhappy no matter what we do. Conversely, the shift may come when times are good but we still lack fulfillment, such as when we have all the money we need but long for another kind of reward, when we have achieved much but still feel empty, or when external recognition isn't sustaining us. These types of challenges motivate us to identify what really matters, and this naturally leads us to rely on internal values.

Our true nature is always aligned with internal values, which include authenticity, compassion, connection, fairness, freedom, inner peace, joy, love, and truth. These, quite simply, are the qualities of spirit. In other words, we don't need to figure out how to create them: they're integral to who we are even if they've been veiled by our conditioning.

When our awareness is tethered to these internal values on a consistent basis we find that our choices, the way we spend our time, and the way we relate to ourselves and others transforms, often quite dramatically.

MORE HEALING FUNDAMENTALS

hen we're dedicated to discovering our authentic selves, the habits of deep healing emerge naturally because they're written in the very fabric of our beings. Every soul is encoded with

Embrace Comfort and Discomfort

information about how to best take care of the body in which it's being housed. Our body and souls truly have very basic needs and from what I've observed, we often make our healing plans far more complicated than they need to be and forget the fundamentals.

A Plant Analogy

A gardener knows that her plants needs certain essential things to thrive: water, the right amount of sun, rich soil, the ongoing addition of organic matter, an environment that is welcoming to beneficial birds and insects, pruning in some cases, possibly shelter from strong winds, and more.

If the plant is missing even one of these things, there is a failure to thrive fully. Great soil doesn't help a plant that gets no water. You won't get as much out of the compost that you're feeding your plants if they need full sun but have been planted in the shade. At the same time when the gardener sees her relationship with her plants as dynamic and mutually growthful, she will intuitively be drawn to practices that enable her plants to thrive.

Similarly, when we stay open to receiving what our body and soul require for our deep healing, we will be led intuitively to the various components that need our attention. As we incorporate these into our lives, we reap more and more benefits.

Eating nourishing food, meditating, eliminating toxins that threaten our health—all are tried and true practices. In addition, common sense tells us that we benefit from clean air and water, community involvement, exposure to nature and sunshine, regular exercise, and spiritual connection. Following is more information about these and other factors that can contribute to an effective formula for deep healing.

Clean Water

Unless you have access to clean spring water, it would be wise to purify your drinking and bathing water to remove chlorine and chemicals.

Chlorine reacts with other chemicals in water to form carcinogens, and it also destroys the beneficial bacteria in our bodies that we depend on for health. Most water, including city water, well water, and spring water, contains over a thousand different chemicals from agricultural and industrial runoff. Our bodies have enough work to do without having to deal with these harmful compounds.

There are many drinking water filtration systems on the market today, and an array of shower and bath filters are also available. In addition to filtering your water, you can take steps to help heal the planet's precious water supply. For example, conserve water at every opportunity and avoid pouring chemicals down the drain.

Community and Connections

As we mature spiritually, we come to realize that all life is interconnected. So, in that sense, being part of your community is the inevitable consequence of being alive. However, deep healing is also about literally being involved in what's happening right where you live. For example, get to know your neighbors; when they need it, lend a helping hand. Shop at the farmers' market and support local businesses; become acquainted with the farmers and business owners. And finally, volunteer to organize community events or be a part of community projects.

The world's longest-lived and healthiest populations have several things in common, including some behaviors you would expect, such as healthy eating and regular exercise. One additional commonality might surprise you: all report having a deep sense of connection and commitment to their extended families and communities. Although most of them have very little in terms of material possessions, these people have the great fortune to know from experience that they can count on those around them in times of need and as they age. Although this kind of security is no longer typical in many modern societies, fostering reciprocal relationships with your family (or family of choice) throughout your lifetime can increase you own sense of security.

Creativity, Talents and Other Gifts

The soul often expresses itself in the world through creative expression. Allowing authentic impulses to flow through our bodies in the form of painting, music, singing, poetry, writing, dancing, cooking, gardening, woodwork, decorating, clothing, and more, is one of the most beautiful, rewarding and inspiring reflections of our divinity in action.

We also each have a unique essence that expresses itself through the talents we have been given. However, we sometimes tend to take our own natural gifts and abilities for granted and don't realize how inspiring they are to others. On the other hand, the people around us may not appreciate our talents, possibly because they don't perceive them to have any monetary worth, so we may become discouraged and decide not to nurture our skills. This scenario is regrettable because using our gifts is thoroughly satisfying for our souls and necessary for our health and happiness. When we nurture and use our special abilities, we enrich not only ourselves but also our families, friends, and communities.

Fresh Air

Get outside and breathe deeply! The air indoors has been shown to be about four times more toxic than the air outdoors. Sources of indoor pollution include building materials, carpets, cleaning products, dust, mold, and upholstery. One way to clear the air is to open the windows regularly, especially when you sleep at night, and to bring plants into the house as well as onto your property to filter the air.

Movement

Every healthy child loves to move, but as adults we tend to forget how satisfying physical activity can be. Besides having sedentary jobs, many of us have been programmed to believe that certain forms of exercise are better than others, or we've forced ourselves to do soulless and mindless forms of exercise that take the fun out of it. In addition, if we've been inactive for awhile, once we do initiate exercise there is an initial stirring up of stagnant emotions which can tend to subconsciously deter us from making movement a habit. Bring awareness to this and do what you can to support your emotional health. At the same time, keep moving every day.

One simple and effective strategy is to move the way you love to move. Think about the activities you've enjoyed throughout your life and can continue to do now. It helps to list a variety of activities to choose from, such as bicycling, canoeing, dancing, fitness classes, gardening, hiking, housework, in-line skating, qigong, skiing, tai chi, and yoga. Don't think of movement as something that has to wait until leisure time; incorporate it into your daily routine by walking or bicycling to work or other local destinations when possible.

Nature

We're deeply nourished by the sights, smells, sounds, and vibrations of nature. Since time immemorial, the natural world has subtly but powerfully taught us the principles of living in balance, harmony, and peace. Today, modern research confirms that "nature therapy" has significant, positive effects on stress and disease that greatly surpass those of drugs and many other forms of therapy. It's gratifying when science confirms what many cultures and individuals have known intuitively for ages.

To take advantage of nature's power to heal, try to get outdoors or connect with nature every day. For example, enjoy a meal outside, go for a walk in a local park, grow some of your own food, or spend your leisure time outdoors. If you can't go to nature, bring nature to you by using plants and other natural objects, such as branches, feathers, flowers, and stones, to decorate your home. Allow yourself to receive and be nourished by the gifts of nature that are all around you.

Prayer

Prayer requires us to dive deep into our hearts and inquire into our most profound longings and aspirations. This in and of itself is intensely revealing. Through the simple practice of prayer we're able to divine what we really want from life. We can then ask for help—from angels, God, or our spiritual guides or masters—in any way that feels comfortable. Once we've spoken our prayers, we need only be open to receiving the outcome. This includes letting go of personal and fear-based agendas and expectations. In addition to helping us identify what we want, prayers can also make us aware of what we're most grateful for. In this way, prayers of thanksgiving can also boost healing.

Rest

In order to heal from within, the body needs rest. When people are sleep deprived, and many members of our fast-paced society are *profoundly* sleep deprived, the whole body is affected. The lack of rest weakens the endocrine system in particular, which affects our energy levels, hormonal balance, moods, reproductive organs, sleep cycles, sugar and fat metabolism, and weight. Even an exceptionally healthful diet can't offset the effects of chronic weariness. And exercising a tired body only stresses the adrenal glands further.

To get the kind of fulfilling rest that supports deep healing, go to bed early and let yourself wake up naturally when you feel rested; if possible, align your retiring and rising rhythms with the setting and rising of the sun. Remove all electronic devices, including the television, from your sleeping space. Regard your bedroom as a deep-healing sanctuary. Keep it clean and uncluttered, and decorate it in a way that feels welcoming and relaxing.

Sunshine

Since the beginning of time human beings and all life have been evolving under the sun's light, warmth and energy which provide a wealth of healing benefits. Many holistic practitioners encourage gentle sunbathing to reverse various health conditions, including acne, cancer, candida, depression, eczema, and psoriasis. Research has shown that sunlight decreases blood pressure and cholesterol, enhances the blood's ability to carry oxygen, increases white blood cell counts to boost immunity, increases growth and height in children, and destroys harmful bacteria to heal infection. In addition, the sun is our greatest source of vitamin D (our bodies synthesize vitamin D when we're exposed to sunlight), which increases metabolism, protects the brain from aging and dementia, strengthens bones and teeth, and supports the immune system.

There are countless ways to get more sunshine, such as sitting outside with your face to the sun while you enjoy breakfast, lunch, or dinner. Or doing a series of sun salutations in a sunny spot in your backyard or a local park, or taking a refreshing outdoor nap in the late afternoon with as much of your skin exposed as possible. Of course, working in your garden or playing outdoors are obvious and very enjoyable ways to naturally bask in the sunlight we all depend on. When you're out in the sun, feel it penetrating deep into the areas of your body that need healing.

Listen to your body's craving for the sun. Use your own experience and common sense to determine how much exposure is safe for you rather than capitulate to media warnings about how "bad" the sun is for you. If the sun is uncomfortable, then it's a good sign that you should be protecting yourself, and there are many methods that work quite well. For example, spend time outdoors when the sun's rays aren't as intense, such as in the early morning or late afternoon. On cooler days in the fall, winter, or spring, find sunny spots that are protected from the wind.

When you need to block direct sun, wear a hat and a long-sleeve shirt and pants made from a light fabric. Avoid using sunscreen unless absolutely necessary; many contain toxic chemicals, although some brands are made with natural ingredients and are worth seeking out if you must spend long periods outside.

The preceding section is meant to help you confirm the positive things that you are already doing for your body and soul, or to help you identify certain components of deep healing that you may be ready to incorporate in your life. Please don't use it as a measuring stick or an "ideal" to live up to, and don't rely on discipline to get there. As mentioned previously, if deep healing is what you're here to do, your own formula will emerge over time and you will naturally find yourself discovering and incorporating activities, practices, and attitudes that your body and soul love.

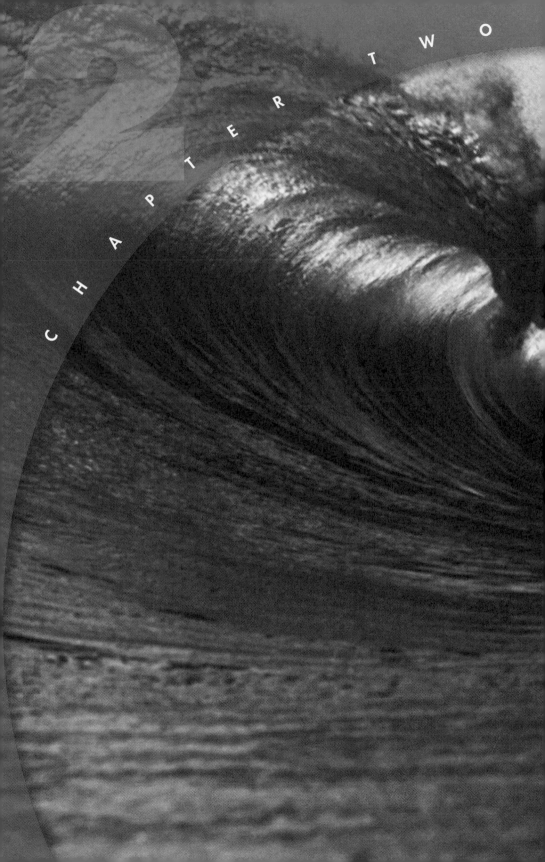

CHAPTER TWO

Good Vibrations

To enter the forest of adventure you must go in
at the point that is darkest, for if there is a way or a path,
it is someone else's.

JOSEPH CAMPBELL

All matter, including you and me, is made of energy. And beyond you and me, a vast dynamic energy field, like a matrix, connects all life. In addition, we're affected by the energy, or vibrations, around us all the time, whether we're aware of it or not. These realizations profoundly affected my view of healing and life in general, and their understanding is a cornerstone to the deep healing journey.

As energy beings, we were all born with our own creative impulse. It's this impulse that sets our lives in motion, and it's this impulse that drives us to fulfill and express ourselves completely. When we resist the unique flow of the energy impulse that we are, we create tension and suffering. When we follow the flow, we experience creativity, health, joy, and peace.

Over time, all energy changes and evolves. Some forms, such as a thought, are relatively short-lived, while others, such as a sea turtle, live much longer. Eventually all energy returns back to where it came from, a place I refer to as pure consciousness.

Unhealthy energy, as we'll see later, can get caught in circular patterns and stagnate, which interferes with our physical well-being and our spiritual evolution. Because true healing is essentially a process of surrendering to the energy flow of your fundamental nature, it's important to understand the properties of energy. When you do, you'll be better equipped to bring awareness to the energy blocks that prevent you from being your authentic self (see chapter 3, page 21) and living the most vibrant life possible.

EVERYTHING IS MADE OF ENERGY AND IT'S ALIVE

From the scientific discipline of quantum physics comes the now fairly common knowledge that there is nothing solid about our world at all. When we go into physical matter deeply enough, we begin to see that amidst the atoms, the building blocks of our universe, are yawning chasms of "empty" space.

Furthermore, scientists have observed that the components of atoms—electrons, protons, and neutrons—seem to flash in and out of existence. Energy in nature, including the energy that makes up a healthy body, is in constant motion: contracting, expanding, flowing, pulsating, radiating, and spiraling in a perpetual dance. So by discovering what happens on the atomic level, we learn one of the biggest lessons of all: what seems solid, still, and immutable is, in fact, not.

Everything in our world, inanimate as well as animate, is made of energy. An apple, a dog, a human being, a pen, a plastic container, a stone, water—all are fundamentally energy, and each has a unique energy pattern and frequency. We perceive these things as solid because they're formed by relatively condensed energy that we can detect with our five senses. Similarly, we can consider that that the space *between* objects is also dynamic, alive, and made of energy. A term often used to describe this energy is "vibration."

Vibrations Are All Around Us

Whether we're aware of it or not, we're constantly picking up the vibrations around us. The vibration of one object affects another, and this phenomenon is called harmonic inductance, or entrainment. As you become more aware of energy, you'll also become increasingly adept at detecting subtle sensations in your body that change with different circumstances. For example, spending time in nature may make you feel relaxed and open, whereas being around negative people may make you feel heavy and sluggish.

Children and animals are particularly sensitive to the energies around them. When we're anxious and upset, for example, children can sense our emotions and will mirror them. Similarly, when we're calm and grounded, our children and pets follow suit.

Thoughts and Emotions Are Also Energy

Thoughts are formless energy that can travel instantly through space and be detected by the objects of our thoughts. If this seems a little farfetched, consider this: We've probably all had the experience of thinking about someone we haven't spoken to in a while and then bumping into

It's Also Deep Feeling

A foundational awareness practice for deep healing is to bring awareness to the subtle energy sensations in your body as you respond to the world around you. This isn't a thoroughly unfamiliar concept. Many of us already pick up unseen "positive" or "negative" energies, or vibes, in the places we visit. For example, notice the subtle sensations in your body when you walk into a church or garden. How do these compare to the sensations you experience when entering a mall or fast-food restaurant? Where in your body do you feel flow and where do you feel blocked?

them or hearing from them out of the blue. Or we call a relative who was just picking up the phone to call us. In addition, we can often get a sense of what kind of day our partners and children are having just by thinking about them. We also have all probably had the experience of having a thought, sharing it with a friend, and finding they were just thinking the same thing. This likely happens more often than we know because we don't share everything that we're thinking. Thoughts may also reach unknown people at a distance, which may explain why groundbreaking discoveries are sometimes made simultaneously by unrelated scientists working at opposite ends of the globe.

Emotions are also energy, and many of us are also aware that we can detect emotional energy. For example, a person might smile when talking to you, but your body may be picking up an entirely different story.

Each human emotion carries a distinct energetic signature that is commonly felt in various places in the body. For example, for many, sadness is felt as heaviness in the chest, while anger is often felt as tightness just below the rib cage. Worry can manifest as constriction in the throat, and joy is felt as lightness and spaciousness throughout the body.

Food is Energy Too

As a nutritionist I love to underscore the fact that food is energy too. Every whole food contains an energy signature that is unique to that food, like a personality. In addition, the food is affected by the energies that it was exposed to during its growth and processing because of harmonic inductance.

For example, when we eat the milk, eggs, or flesh of land and sea animals that have suffered, endured violence, and been frustrated and sad during their lives, we take in that energy when we consume these foods. Because most of us are so far removed from the source of our food today, we don't see the countless ways these innocent animals are mistreated and tortured. Still, their distress reaches us: The eggs, meat, and milk we con-

Food and Emotions

Food is an emotional topic, tied to memories, traditions, and many other aspects of life. So when you read about food in this book, you're likely to find yourself reacting one way or another—in agreement, perhaps, or with skepticism about new ideas. For example, when you read about food animals, do you feel tension? If so, where do you feel it? You may be sensing areas of trapped energy related to your own energy body as well as the collective energy body (including that of the animals).

To tune in more fully, keep your belly soft, your shoulders relaxed, and your heart open. Bring your awareness to the sensations you're feeling without judgment and notice what happens. We'll explore how this can free blocked energy in Chapter 3.

sume are awash with their painful emotions and fear. Is it any wonder, then, that antidepressants are so commonly prescribed these days? Or that crime, violence, and suicide are on the rise?

Although industrialized agriculture provides much of the food now available in North America, there are still independent farmers and organic farmers who honor their connection with the earth. They do so by growing food that is nourishing and clean, and they infuse the food they grow with love and wholesomeness. When we select and prepare food with sincere blessings of wholeness and peace for ourselves and our families, we become saturated with the food's positive energy.

By understanding this, we come to see that food is much more than mere calories, minerals, proteins, and vitamins. The emotions, intentions, and values that we bring to the cultivation and preparation of our food affect us immensely in unseen but very real ways.

The Frequency of Health and Disease

If everything is made of energy, then theoretically, everything can be measured according to the frequency of its energy waves. In reality, many researchers have discovered ways to measure the frequency of the human body. Although every cell, tissue, and organ has its own resonance, on average, a human body vibrates at 62 to 68 megahertz (MHz).

Royal Rife, an American inventor, developed a machine that measures frequencies, and he concluded that every disease has a specific frequency. Subsequently, the research of Bruce Tainio, a biologist who founded Tainio Technology (a company that provides natural products and solutions for agriculture and the environment), identified the following relationships between body frequency and illness:

- When a body's frequency drops below 62 MHz, human cells can start to mutate.
- When a body is fighting off a cold or flu, the body's frequency is 58 MHz.
- When candida is present, the body's frequency is 55 MHz.
- When the Epstein-Barr virus is present, the body's frequency is 52 MHz.
- When a body's frequency drops to 42 MHz, cancer can appear.
- When the death process begins, the body's frequency has been measured at 20 MHz.

It's clear that pathogens and diseased cells thrive at specific suboptimal frequencies, and good vibrations are crucial for good health and deep healing. In acknowledgment of the fact that health is only possible when energy is flowing, most holistic therapies—including acupuncture, homeopathy, Reiki, and yoga—focus on moving stuck and low-vibration energies (which also may be referred to by other names, such as chi or prana, in various healing traditions).

The condition and frequency of the physical body aren't the only determinants of health. In fact, our mental and emotional states can also profoundly affect our energy frequencies, as can our spiritual connection. For example, a negative mental and emotional state has been shown to lower a person's frequency by 10 to 12 MHz. Conversely, meditation, prayer, and other positive states can raise it by 10 to 15 MHz.

INTUITION CAN GUIDE DEEP HEALING

When we become more aware of the energy body, we become open to the various ways in which it communicates with us about healing. These messages can be instant or delayed and can come in the form of dreams, images, new ideas or interests, specific guidance, or words.

Once you've committed to your healing, and begun to turn your awareness to areas of blocked energy, you may find, as I did, that you'll sometimes hear about a course or retreat, and something inside you will light up. There are many courses, teachers, and practitioners in the holistic health world, and while many have value, your intuition can help you discern which are most appropriate for your particular journey.

Many other fairly common experiences are actually your intuition speaking to you. For example, when you meet certain people, you may just know, with your whole being, that you need to spend time with them or learn from them. Or when you go to the market, you're strongly

Intuitive Messages and Guidance

Think back to a time when you "just knew" something. How did that feel in your body? Were you able to immediately trust this feeling, or did you need to run it through your brain first? Be open to trusting intuitive messages. Better yet, ask a question and then wait for the answer to come in the form of intuitive guidance.

drawn to certain foods and turned off by others for no apparent reason. When you wake up in the morning, certain tasks might "light up" on your mental to-do list. Or when you're having a conversation, some words or gestures might feel more alive than others.

Similarly, subtle shifts can indicate when you're receiving messages from your energy body. You may develop new interests in health-related topics or begin to see certain things with fresh eyes. For example, a book that's been on your shelf for years may suddenly draw your notice. Or you may find that you begin to enjoy certain activities, such as cooking or exercise, that felt like dull chores in the past.

As you begin to be guided by intuition, you may lose interest in activities or things that once brought you pleasure. Many of your inauthentic ways of being will gradually fall away, and you'll be more likely to be open to new possibilities. When you're willing to listen to the energy body, you begin to communicate directly with your soul in subtle but powerful ways. Whether you count on the deepest power within yourself or rely on an external power, such as the universe, God, or another divinity, rest assured that this positive force delights in your healing and is helping you in countless ways. It's up to you to be open—*to listen deeply*—by learning to be silent and still, listening to your body, letting go of control, and surrendering to the mystery of your unfolding.

The Energetic Yes

Once we set our intention to heal deeply and learn to tune in to energy sensations in the body, we begin to notice what I call the energetic yes. You've no doubt already experienced an energetic yes even if you didn't think of it in those terms. In essence, it's the sudden feeling you get when you resonate positively with a new idea, person, or other stimulus. You might associate it with intuition, but it's a specific kind of knowing: the physical response you have when someone or something really "clicks" with you.

An energetic yes can feel different for different people, so it's important to identify how your body communicates an energetic yes to you. It may simply feel like a light going on inside you or a slight rise in aliveness or awareness. It could also feel like an opening of the heart or a surge of warmth to the hands, feet, and other parts of the body. Some people report that they feel tingling, commonly just on one side of the body and often on the right side. And sometimes, an energetic yes manifests as sudden tears in response to something that your hear, read, or see.

The energetic yes is one of the primary ways our soul communicates with us. When you start recognizing it in your life, you'll find it occurs with greater and greater frequency.

The Chakras

The ancient yoga-based chakra system provides an excellent map for getting to know the energy body. Becoming aware of your chakras, the major energy centers of the body, is helpful in deep healing because blocked chakras can contribute to illness. Paying attention to your chakras can be an effective aspect of your healing intuition.

The human body has seven main energy centers, which align vertically along the center of the body. Chakra energy radiates in all directions, but the middle five chakras radiate primarily to the front and back. The remaining two chakras are the base chakra and the crown chakra; the base chakra extends strongly down toward the earth and the crown chakra extends strongly up toward the heavens. The individual chakras bring the life force to specific body parts, communicate intuitive information to us, and correlate to common life and spiritual lessons.

Following are brief descriptions of each chakra, including its location and function. As you read through this section, notice how the different parts of your body feel in response to the information.

ROOT CHAKRA. Found at the base of the spine, the root chakra relates to feelings of belonging and support; its primary goal is having our basic physical needs met. It's responsible for the health of the adrenal glands, bones, feet, legs, and rectum.

SACRAL CHAKRA. Found between the pubic bone and the navel, the sacral chakra relates to finding harmony and balance in relationships as well as tapping into our creativity. It's responsible for the health of the colon, ovaries, prostate, small intestine, testes, and uterus.

SOLAR PLEXUS CHAKRA. Found above the navel and below the rib cage, the solar plexus chakra helps us uncover our personal power and authentic values, or in other words, it helps us to separate from the tribe. It's responsible for the health of much of the digestive system, including the gallbladder, kidneys, liver, pancreas, and stomach.

DEEP HEALING
The Chakras

Sahasrara

Ajna

Vishuddha

Anahata

Manipura

Swadhisthana

Muladhara

Crown chakra

Brow chakra

Throat chakra

Heart chakra

Solar Plexus chakra

Sacral chakra

Root chakra

HEART CHAKRA. Found in the middle of the chest at the level of the arm-pits, the heart chakra focuses on unconditional self-love. It's responsible for the health of the arms, breasts, hands, heart, lungs, and thymus gland.

THROAT CHAKRA. Found at the base of the throat in the sternal notch, the throat chakra is primarily oriented toward authentic self-expression and surrendering to the song of the soul. It's responsible for the health of the ears, jaw, neck, teeth, and thyroid gland.

BROW CHAKRA. The brow chakra is found in the center of the forehead. It helps us to see beyond conditioning and know truth.

CROWN CHAKRA. The crown chakra is found on the top of the head. As our spiritual connector, it helps us to experience ourselves as spiritual beings and to communicate with the spiritual realms.

The last two chakras also work as a team. Both the brow and crown chakras are responsible for the health of the brain, the eyes, and the pineal and pituitary glands.

When you sit in stillness, spend a minute or so tuning in to each chakra. Simply be present. Pay attention to anything that arises, including emotions, images, memories, and sensations. Take note of any guidance that comes to you.

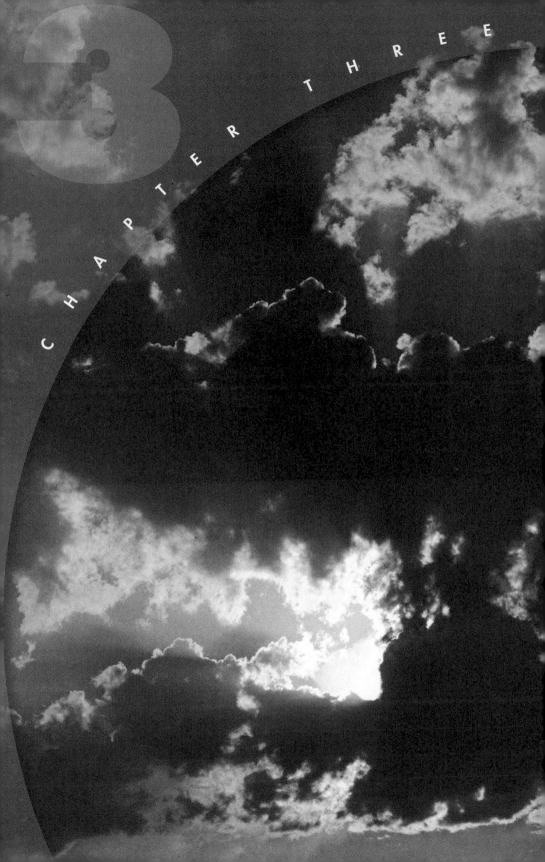

Freeing the Energy Body

At the core of the false self is a void of deficiency derived from an essential turning away from one's own divinity, either out of natural development, despair, or simply by succumbing to the trance of the world with all its masks of deception and harsh obligation to conform to its insanity.

ADYASHANTI

In order to free the energy body, it's helpful to understand how energy gets blocked over the course of our lives. We are then more willing and able to bring awareness to lower vibration pockets in our being. As we *see* through the eyes of presence, disidentification with the circumstances, beliefs, and emotions related to these energy blockages happens automatically. The energy is then free to follow its inherent intelligence, which is always aligned with our highest potential.

Healing Energy Flow Is Happening Through You Always

Of primary importance is the understanding that energy need not be manipulated, as it is already coursing through you with the intelligence of your essential self. The stream of energy called Life is flowing through each one of us, and our ability to enjoy and benefit from it depends on how much we surrender to it. The process of deep healing is not about searching or trying to create energy flow, but rather primarily about discovering where we block Life from flowing and accessing the attitude that dissolves these blockages.

Where Energy Blockages Come From

Although we're influenced by the emotions and energy we pick up in the womb, our energy is as clear as it has ever been when we're born. Our earliest experiences begin to form our beliefs about ourselves, others, and the world

21

around us, and these beliefs directly affect our authentic energy impulse. Our unique energy is affected by the specific circumstances we're born into. Naturally, we're influenced by our parents, siblings, and extended family; their societal, political, and religious values; and various demographic and geographic factors.

From the very beginning, the beliefs and emotions we're exposed to may help or hinder our ability to develop the authentic aspects of ourselves. Typically, the people in our lives don't think in terms of how they can help us become who and what we truly are. Because of their own conditioning, fears, and lack of awareness, our caregivers, teachers, and other community members unconsciously set up roadblocks all around our authentic selves. In addition, they tend to shape us into people much like themselves. This makes them comfortable and ensures that we fit in. Ultimately, many of us lose our authentic selves through conditioning and adopt the false beliefs we're exposed to.

ENERGY AND THE CONDITIONED SELF

The conditioned self is the doorway to deep healing. The complex of inauthentic beliefs and stuck emotions that has been created since the beginning of our lives affects our way of seeing the world and being in the world so that we're no longer relating to life from a true place. Our conditioning leads us to act in ways that temporarily keep us safe, such as not being true to ourselves in order to make others comfortable, trying to be perfect to get approval from others, shying away from intimacy to avoid being seen or getting hurt, taking care of others at our own expense, hiding our emotions to avoid being shamed, not asking for what we need in order to avoid rejection, controlling others to protect our vulnerability, not drawing attention to ourselves to avoid judgment from others, and avoiding challenges to keep failure at bay.

Disowning or feeling ashamed of our inauthentic patterns is not the way to heal them, however. In fact, the opposite is true. We need to acknowledge, accept, and even love these parts of ourselves in order to liberate all of the energy that is being tied up in them.

ENERGY AND FALSE BELIEFS

To recapture who we really are, we must be able to recognize and accept that we've been subjected to conditioning and false beliefs, particularly during our early years. However, we tend to push these beliefs and their associated emotions and energy patterns outside of our awareness; I call this the "shadow side" of ourselves. When we can't recognize or acknowledge false beliefs, we're unable to see how they affect our worldview and our health.

DEEP HEALING

The Gifts

When you begin to question stressful beliefs and open to your entire emotional experience, the true expression of your unconditioned being effortlessly shines through:

- The energy body is freed up, allowing for deep physical healing and soul-guided living.
- Talents and abilities that you were previously unaware of, and that you will thoroughly enjoy, surface.
- More and more aspects of your life and lifestyle, including friends, hobbies, intimate relationships, leisure activities, service, and work, begin to line up with your true nature.
- Your presence positively affects and inspires those around you.
- Your level of consciousness increases. You look at life from an expanded perspective and approach challenges with inner stability so that evolution is ongoing. You become what spiritual teacher Thomas Huebl calls a "continuous living update of yourself."
- You see and act on solutions to planetary problems that weren't available to you from previous levels of conditioning.

"I'M INSIGNIFICANT." When caregivers don't allow children to explore the world with a reasonable amount of freedom, or when children lose ongoing power struggles to adults, they may come to believe that they're unimportant or that they'll never have control over their lives. This eventual dull acquiescence may mask deep and lingering anger and can inhibit creativity, motivation, and willpower later in life.

"I'M NOT GOOD ENOUGH." When caregivers don't teach children healthy ways of competing, children may come to feel that they don't measure up, either in comparison to their peers or in accordance with adults' expectations. If children aren't encouraged to better themselves for the sheer fun of exploring their potential, they can begin to feel like they're not good enough, especially if they're pressured to win at all costs or receive praise only when they succeed. The sense of falling short of expectations can continue beyond childhood. Many adults judge themselves harshly, compare themselves to others, and experience deep feelings of dissatisfaction. These behaviors and emotions are most likely to surface during times of stress.

"I'M NOT LOVABLE." Most parents, to greater or lesser extents, are unable to fully express unconditional love for their children, because they don't fully love themselves. In the mildest form, it can manifest as emotional distance. It can also involve shaming children, or even verbally or physically abusing them. Self-hatred begins to set in and can affect their ability to go out into the world with openness and confidence.

"IT'S NOT OKAY TO FEEL." Children are very sensitive and quite adept at picking up on adult emotions and energies. When caregivers suppress and distort certain emotions, this can be very confusing for children. For example, when a child senses anger from a parent, but the parent shows affection or otherwise acts in a way that belies anger, the child can learn to fear or suppress emotion. The same outcome can occur if a child senses an emotion but the parent diminishes it, especially by denying the emotion and shaming the child.

"THERE'S SOMETHING WRONG WITH ME." It's not uncommon for parents to create idealized versions of their children and imagine that the children have certain ways of behaving, being, communicating, and thinking. Children can pick up on these unrealistic expectations. Because children want nothing more than to please the people they depend on, they'll begin to drop some of their authentic ways and adopt behaviors that will get them praise and attention. They begin to believe (like the parents, in fact) that there is something wrong with them that needs to be fixed. When these children grow to adulthood, they may become perfectionists or people-pleasers. They're also likely to feel disconnected from their true selves and experience the discomfort that comes with not being who they really are.

"THERE'S NEVER ENOUGH." When caregivers aren't able to consistently meet children's needs because they're caught in their own emotions, the children don't receive the presence and attention they need to thrive. Driven by guilt, the parents may then shower the children with attention, food, toys, or treats. When children have this experience of feast or famine, in later life they may experience a neediness that can't be satisfied. This can lead to addictive behaviors, which are extremely draining for the affected individuals as well as the people around them.

Because these beliefs become fixed, they continue to color the lens through which we view our lives right into adulthood. We are often no longer responding to life from our true nature but from a false self that has been conditioned by its experiences. When a relationship ends, we might interpret it as a confirmation that we're unlovable. When our child struggles, we might see it as our own failure. When we are unable to find a job, we may believe that there's something wrong with us.

ENERGY AND EMOTIONS

 houghts and interpretations create reactions in the body that we call emotions. In addition to being nervous and chemical in nature, "e-motions" are energetic patterns that are meant to be

False Beliefs

As you read about false beliefs, did you notice tension and resistance in your body? You may have felt guilty or sad if you recognized yourself in some of the scenarios, either as a parent or a grown child. The goal of including these scenarios was to promote understanding, not to create despair or blame. The best way to use this information is to identify where blocked energy related to these beliefs has been stored in your body. See if you can give these energies more space to move and free themselves by keeping your belly soft, your shoulders relaxed, and your heart open.

If you're a parent, try to connect with your children energetically and spiritually. Be open to receiving intuitive guidance regarding what they need to nourish all aspects of their being as they grow and mature.

in motion. Everything we have experienced and haven't completely processed leaves an emotional residue in the body that results in blocked or sluggish energy. Blocked energy limits our ability to feel, relate to others, and heal on all levels—emotionally, spiritually, and physically.

Most of us are comfortable with certain emotions and uncomfortable with others. Maybe as children we were told that showing certain emotions was a sign of weakness, or we witnessed our parents holding back their emotions, or we saw adults using addictions to deal with their emotions. We learned to stop ourselves from feeling certain emotions, and as a result these emotions became trapped in our tissues and compromised our health.

In order to keep our emotions flowing and free up blocked areas of the energy field, we need to stop thinking of uncomfortable emotions as "bad" and pleasant emotions as "good." All emotions are potentially valuable messengers of self-knowledge and truth. Grasping at pleasant emotions to avoid the challenging ones is the root of all addictions, not to mention a profoundly soul-numbing way of relating to life. By creating a friendly awareness of all emotions, we're able to free up the tremendous amount of life force used to suppress the uncomfortable ones.

In addition, the gift that comes with setting emotions free is that our capacity to feel all of them is enhanced, particularly their opposite. For example feeling, experiencing and expressing sadness gives us access to our natural capacity to feel more joy. Feeling, experiencing, and expressing anger gives us access to our natural capacity to feel more patience. Feeling, experiencing, and expressing apathy gives us access to the natural capacity to feel motivated. Feeling, experiencing, and expressing fear gives us access to our natural capacity to feel courage. Feeling, experiencing, and expressing boredom gives us access to our natural capacity to feel inspired.

Uncomfortable Emotions

When you experience an uncomfortable emotion, notice where you feel it in your body and open to it with curiosity and kindness. Give it space to exist, and it will dance its way through your system on its own. This may take time or happen almost instantaneously. Adopting an expressive outlet may also be helpful. Creating art, having honest conversations, journaling, listening to music, moving intuitively, and spending time in nature are some activities that may help to free an emotion. When you completely let go of judgment and control, the emotion will be set free and integrated back into pure consciousness.

ENERGY AND RELATIONSHIPS

*E*verything and everyone reflects energy information back to us. When we spend time with people, or even simply think about them, we may notice the energy sensations in our body if we pay close attention. We usually attribute such feelings to something inherent in the other person, particularly if the sensations are unpleasant. We may say, "She has bad energy." Or, "He annoys me." The truth, however, is that our feelings about the other person are simply reflecting our own energies and stuck patterns.

This is the principle of harmonic inductance at work. The energy patterns we perceive as negative in others are the very ones we have ourselves. Otherwise, the impressions we get from someone else wouldn't stick to us; they would simply move through. Every day we're given the gift of being shown, often over and over again, our own unhealthy energy patterns. It's up to us to receive this gift and use it in our own healing.

By accepting this radical self-responsibility, we can also help others to heal. For example, let's say my partner and I both have issues with anger; when one of us gets angry, the other feels it intensely and becomes defensive and angry too. So I decide to focus on anger in my meditation practice. I begin to create the space for anger to appear when I'm sitting in stillness, and I dedicate myself to treating anger as though it were a helpless little kitten sitting in my hand. I open to anger with all the gentleness and kindness I can manage. I welcome anger into my experience and bring more and more awareness to the details of the sensations that come with it. I find the place in me that is truly compassionate in the face of my anger. Then one day, my partner is feeling annoyed. I recognize the energy in the room and in my body, but because I've developed a greater capacity to be still in the face of anger, I don't react as I once did. Instead, I feel compassion for my partner and his humanness. Because the relational space feels safe for my partner, he's able to relax more and more over time and acknowledge what is going on for him.

The Law of Attraction

Energy is governed by the law of attraction. We attract people who have similar emotional and vibrational patterns. We also attract people who reflect back to us our fears and weaknesses as well as our strengths and potential. We attract experiences that we need to help us to grow. We even attract physical challenges, including symptoms and diseases, that can teach us about ourselves and encourage us to let go of energy, thoughts, and emotional patterns that result in inauthentic ways of being. In addition, we draw to us all of the resources, both physical and spiritual, that we need to learn about our true nature and heal in the process.

Of all these influences that we're able to draw to ourselves, our closest relationships hold some of the greatest gifts on the path to deep healing. Because of the law of attraction, we attract people with whom we share common lessons and karma. It is through our relationships that we discover our fears, motivations, strengths, and weaknesses. When we're challenged in our relationships, the common tendency is to blame the other person—to judge, try to control, and insist that *they* change. However, the most transformative attitude is to turn our awareness towards ourselves, particularly where we feel resistance in our energy body, as well as questioning the beliefs that are anchoring these energies in our field.

For example, as a person who is interested in health, you may find yourself frustrated by the way others care (or don't care) for themselves. When you insist that someone you love, such as your child, parent, or partner, take better care of himself, what is actually going on? Is it true that at this particular point in his life—given his past experiences, emotional health, and where he is on his path now—that he should be doing anything different than he currently is? How does it make you feel to hold on to the belief that he should be taking better care of himself? Are you frustrated that he simply keeps doing what he wants to do? If there's tension and discomfort in your body, it's there to tell you that you're fighting with reality. Every person's body, and how he takes care of it, is his business. Your reaction is your business.

Through my own experiences and during conversations with clients, I've been reminded over and over again that when we worry about how others manage their health, we're actually being invited to take a closer look at how we take care of our own health. As we deepen our commitment to greater health, we must inevitably look at the emotions and fear that affect our body-soul relationship. When the body and soul are both healthy and have a healthy relationship, we naturally make choices that continue to support this positive state. When there's a disconnect between body and soul, making the necessary repairs and addressing our own health can be hard work. That's why we choose to avoid our own challenges by focusing on other people's health instead.

One of the greatest causes of human suffering is the habit of creating idealized versions of the people in our lives. We do this with our children, coworkers, friends, parents, partners, and pretty much everyone who is significant to us. We create these fantasies to protect ourselves from our "pain body." This term was coined by author Eckhart Tolle to describe the conditioned self, including its false beliefs and painful emotions. For example, the daughter who believes her father should be less critical hides her own fear and lack of self-worth. The parent who thinks his children should apply themselves to their schoolwork hides his feelings of inadequacy. The woman who believes her partner should be more loving avoids looking at her own self-hatred. And the man who feels his boss should be less demanding avoids his own feelings of insecurity. The truth is that we want people to change not for themselves but for our comfort. It's essential to see that when we've created false ideals of the people in our lives and they don't measure up, and they never will, we suffer. This is why it's so important to question painful beliefs. Only by questioning false beliefs can we let go of them and fall in love with reality. And by falling in love with reality, we lay the foundation for creating peace in our lives.

I've discovered that the more at peace I am with my life, the less I'm inclined to try to control and change the people in it. Instead, I experience a gentle but empowering way of being that trusts in the wisdom of each person's journey. I suspect that this is what Mahatma Gandhi meant when he urged us to be the change that we want to see in the world.

Healing Relationships

I've also discovered that when we're in touch with our energy body, see the world as it truly is, and are at peace with ourselves, we're better at helping others who are suffering. For example, if my friend has cancer, when I sit with her, I can open myself to feeling all of the energies that we share between us, including the fear, frustration, joy, love, and sadness. If I'm not able to be in her physical presence, I can bring her into my mind during my meditation practice and feel how my body responds. I can then create space by giving everything that I feel the right to exist. My friend will receive the benefits of my meditation even if she lives one hundred miles away because energy is not governed by time or space. In addition, when I visit her next, I'll be more present because I won't be struggling with uncomfortable emotions.

Energy awareness is a tool we can use twenty-four hours a day. When combined with meditation (see chapter 4, page 33), it can be the most powerful part of a deep-healing practice. This is true for several reasons. First, we become adept at recognizing energy at work all around us, and we can harness this energy to boost our own vitality. Second, we remove

Awareness is a Powerful Solvent of Blocked Energy

Sitting in the silence of a meditation practice gives us the opportunity to watch the various layers of our conditioning come and go. Over time we begin to discern the difference between what is changing and what always stays the same. Beneath the stories, beliefs, opinions, sensations, emotions and physical issues, is a quiet presence that's untouched by our circumstances. When tension, discomfort and other sensations are brought into our awareness without trying to manipulate them in any way, there is a spaciousness created around blocked energy that sets it in motion. For an example of a guided meditation, see chapter 4, page 33.

harmful tendencies from our shadow side and integrate them into our light side, which is essential for healing. Third, we create the foundation for peaceful relationships that promote mutual growth. Fourth, we help others heal by being present to emotions that they don't yet have the capacity to work through. And finally, we help to clear collective energy patterns by meditating on marginalized aspects of our culture or history, thereby preserving the lessons they hold for us. For example, I'm quite interested in clearing our collective fear of disease. Others have focused on clearing energies around environmental devastation or energies remaining from wars or ethnic cleansing.

ENERGY AND PHYSICAL HEALING

*E*very cell, tissue, and organ in the body needs free-flowing energy to function well. When we hold on to false beliefs, and the unavoidable negative emotions that they anchor in our bodies, energy stagnates and can lead to disease over time. As medical intuitive Carolyn Myss has pointed out, our biography, in fact, becomes our biology.

The stages of symptoms and disease can be viewed from both a physical and energetic standpoint. Even though the physical body and the energy body are one and the same (the physical is simply condensed energy that can be felt, seen, and touched by the senses), it can be helpful to separate the two realms to understand how one leads to the other. The stages of symptoms and disease follow:

STAGE ONE. Because we're essentially energy beings, all symptoms begin on an energetic level, primarily as stagnant emotions that are being anchored by false beliefs. Our energy bodies reflect both individual energies, which are a direct result of our life experiences, and collective energies, which make up the energy "soup" of the society that we live in.

STAGE TWO. An area of contraction is created around the suppressed energy to keep it out of our awareness. We are likely to pull our attention out of our physical body and start living in our minds and "stories."

STAGE THREE. The contraction leads to habitual tension in the surrounding tissues that we are often unaware of.

STAGE FOUR. Tension decreases the inflow of physical resources, such as blood, lymph, nutrients, and oxygen, and energetic resources, also known as chi, the life force, or prana. Tension also decreases the outflow of physical and energetic toxins.

STAGE FIVE. Over time, the lack of flow begins to affect the proper functioning of the physical body. Often, the first sign of disease is fatigue. The physical tissues aren't receiving what they need, and toxins are building up. Also, much of our life force is being tied up in maintaining suppressed energies. During this stage, we often ignore the fatigue and push ourselves to keep up with life.

STAGE SIX. If we don't acknowledge the fatigue, eventually the body will begin to malfunction in subtle ways: we gain weight, our joints feel tight, our digestion is compromised, we have minor skin complaints, we aren't sleeping well, and so on. Modern medical tests don't pick up any issues at this stage.

STAGE SEVEN. If we continue to disregard what the body is asking from us, it will experience greater and greater imbalance. Symptoms will worsen, and medical testing can confirm the presence of a specific disease.

STAGE EIGHT. If we decide to take medication or have a medical procedure, without looking at the mental and emotional causes, it's likely that these options will alleviate some symptoms while creating others, which often leads to another drug or procedure. If the energy body has not been addressed, the root cause of the disease has not been addressed.

When we examine these developmental stages of disease, we can fully appreciate that the wisest course of action is to nip disease in the bud, when it's still just blocked emotional energy. It's also wise to rest when we feel tired, clean up our diet, do a juice fast, and deal with the burden of stress in our lives before we fall ill. But even people who have been diagnosed with a disease can heal by committing to health and peace, giving the body and soul what they need to thrive, and opening to receive all the help that is available. Remember though that because the physical body is made of the densest energy, it will take longer than the mind and emotions to heal. For example, once you've begun to release the frustration and anger that is contributing to arthritis, know that it will usually take more time for the body to complete the healing on the physical level, so be patient.

The table below lists several disease states and the emotions that may contribute to them. If you have one of these conditions, you might consider turning your awareness to the body to uncover the false beliefs and emotions that could be affecting your health. When you do, the resulting spiritual lessons can support more positive states of being and improved vitality.

Please note that what is being offered is simply a starting point. If you have one of these conditions, you might consider turning your awareness to the body to uncover the false beliefs and emotions that could be affecting your health. When you do, the resulting spiritual lessons can support more positive states of being and improved vitality.

BLOCKED ENERGY AND DISEASE STATES

Symptom	Mental/emotional pattern	Spiritual lesson
AIDS	Self-rejection, attacking oneself	Self-love, acceptance
Asthma	Feeling smothered	Giving ourselves space to breathe
Brain diseases	Over-reliance on thought and conditioned interpretation	Connecting with intuition
Breast cancer	Resentment around nurturing others	Self-care
Colitis	Anger (especially toward family members) turned inward	Setting healthy boundaries
Constipation	The inability to let go, not feeling at home	Being at home with our feelings
Diabetes	The inability to take in the sweetness of life	Feeling worthy of goodness
Excessive fat	Layers of protection, sensitivity to criticism	Self-acceptance, joyful expression
Eye issues	Being lost in illusion	Being willing to see the truth
Gallstones	Unexpressed anger, buildup of toxic emotions	Softening around anger, expression through creativity
Heart disease	A lack of connection with the soul	Listening to and following the heart
High blood pressure	Hidden secrets and shame	Being honest with ourselves
Kidney stones	Unexpressed fear	Accessing courage by acknowledging fear
Migraines	Painful thoughts	Questioning beliefs
PMS	Suppressing emotions, power struggles in relationships	Taking time to be still, feeling and expressing authentically
Prostate disease	Blocked creativity	Letting go of inauthentic ways of being
Thyroid issues	Fighting the way things are	Surrendering to the natural flow of life

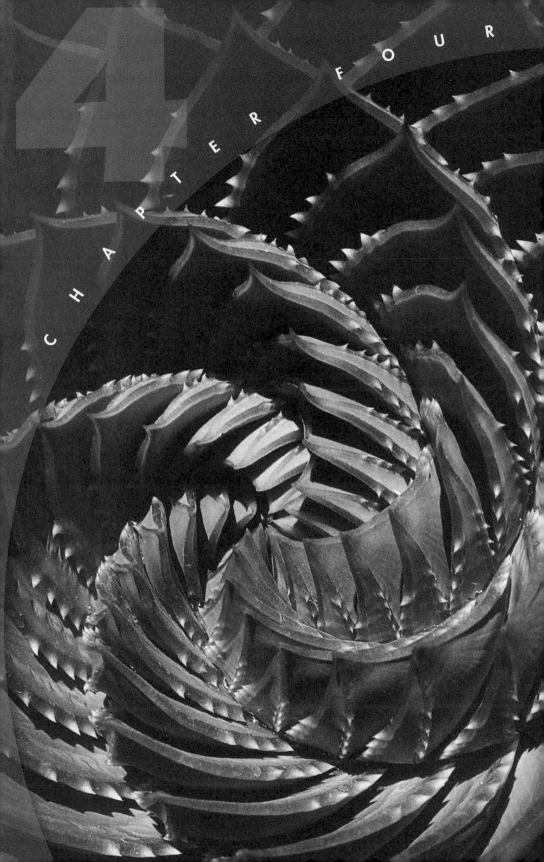

Spirituality and Meditation

The joy of Being, which is the only true happiness, cannot come to you through any form, possession, achievement, person, or event—through anything that happens. That joy cannot come to you—ever. It emanates from the formless dimension within you, from consciousness itself and thus is one with who you are.

ECKHART TOLLE

When we come to understand the roles of energy and spirit in our lives, we desire to be more aware, be more awake, and delve more deeply into consciousness. We know instinctively that the ever-changing surface of life that we see, like the ocean waves, conceals depths that are constant, still, and timeless. Here lies the unchanging self and truth; connecting to this place is the foundation of deep healing. In the precious moments of stillness and silence we are nourished by our souls.

MEDITATION IS THE TRUE SOURCE OF HEALING

Regular meditation is a core practice in many, if not most, spiritual traditions. Through meditation, we leave behind surface events and arrive at the deepest place available to us. Eventually, we never leave. This is called enlightenment, which simply means that our physical self is completely and consistently infused with our true spiritual nature.

While there are many different meditation practices, true meditation is not a practice but rather our natural state. When we sit in stillness, we aren't creating a meditative state. Instead, we're falling gently into what is our natural way of being.

Deep healing requires that we recognize our spiritual selves and address our spiritual needs, just as we attend to our physical and emotional needs. "Spiritual" pertains to spirit, the vitalizing force in each one of us. To be spir-

Spiritual Support

Although the spiritual component of deep healing is a personal journey, you can take advantage of many sources of support and guidance along the way:

- A spiritual practice involves setting aside time on a daily basis to deeply listen to your heart and body through meditation.

- A spiritual guide or teacher is someone you trust and resonate with. Choose a teacher who has walked a path that inspires you and can make the process of deep healing clearer and shorter, particularly by helping you when you're stuck.

- A spiritual retreat provides the opportunity to spend time away from your regular daily routine and distractions. Periodic retreats allow you to tap ever more deeply into your core essence.

- A spiritual community is a group of like-minded people who value soul-centered living.

- Books, courses, and other resources about spirituality can introduce you to new perspectives.

- Spiritual friends are close friends with whom we can share our experiences and who appreciate our efforts toward living a more awake life.

itual, we need not be religious or identify with one specific organized religion or deity. In fact, just the opposite is true: because we all possess spirit, we are all spiritual beings, regardless of religious affiliation.

Most people on a spiritual path describe their quest as one of awareness and awakening. The highly individualistic journey of deep healing incorporates spiritual lessons all along the way. For example, when we can bring them into our awareness, even the physical symptoms of illness and detoxification provide spiritual lessons. The key to spiritual awareness, like the key to deep healing itself, is learning how to listen to yourself. One of the most effective ways to listen is through a deep-healing meditation, and a sample meditation is provided in this chapter (see page 36).

DEEP-HEALING MEDITATION TIPS

*T*rue meditation requires that you let go of the external details, feelings, sensations, and thoughts that constantly arise in the conditioned mind. All you need to do is sit quietly for five minutes to experience this for yourself. Release all surface phenomena simply by allowing them to be as they are. Manipulate nothing; resist nothing. Just sit quietly, completely relinquish control, and rest as pure awareness. You'll begin to sense the eternal, spacious, and sweet essence of your own true nature, which is formless, unchanging, and untouched by circumstances, space, and time.

When you engage in body-centered meditation, a part of you remains untouched and unaffected by the outer world. The still presence that is gazing out from behind your eyes is the same as it was the day you were born. It's the very source of awareness that holds your true nature. Inherent in it are the qualities of faith, oneness, peace, truth, and wisdom.

It's possible to shine awareness on the surface details of your moments at the same time as you rest in awareness itself. The following tips provide elaboration and can be useful when you practice the deep-healing meditation on page 36.

Sit in a Comfortable Position

When you sit in meditation, it's very helpful to get into a position that will create long-term comfort. This can be in a chair or on a bench, couch, or meditation pillow. While true meditation is available no matter how your body is aligned, you can remain more engaged in a vibrant meditation session when your posture is supportive and your muscles are relaxed. Under these conditions, the energy body flows more easily.

Wherever you're sitting, position your pelvis so that your lumbar spine, which is in your lower back, curves naturally. Start by dropping your pubic bone until you're sitting right on top of the sitz bones, which are the pointy bones in your buttocks. Avoid tucking your tailbone under your body or resting on the back of the sitz bones. This will level off your pelvis and allow your lower back to curve as it should. Then position your chin so it's parallel to the floor and slide your neck back until your ears are over your shoulders. Sitting in this position will prevent your head from jutting forward and creating strain on the neck and upper back muscles. This position also will prevent your body from collapsing forward, which hinders breathing and digestion. You should feel as though your collar bones are lengthening outward and allowing your chest to expand. Finally, you should feel your tailbone extending down toward the earth and the crown of your head extending up to the heavens.

By the way, it's best not to lie down during meditation since your body will relax and you're likely to fall asleep. Even if you stay awake, your meditation experience may be quite dull. The idea is for your body to be relaxed and engaged simultaneously during meditation; the inner experience should be awake and alive.

Close Your Eyes

True meditation can be done with eyes closed or open. This deep-healing meditation requires you to bring your awareness to your inner world, and for many people this is easier with eyes closed and without the distraction of visual images. Some meditation practices encourage

DEEP HEALING
A Meditation

The following meditation is for healing the body. For more in-depth guidance, see pages 33 to 39.

Sit in a comfortable position. Close your eyes. Allow your belly to soften in its own time. Allow your breath to deepen in its own way. Bring your attention to your breath, both near your nose and in your body. Do this over and over until your mind begins to be less dominant.

Begin to notice other sensations in your body. Gently turn your awareness to both comfortable and uncomfortable sensations. Now think of a health condition you want to heal. Notice how your body feels when you bring this condition into your awareness. Draw your attention to the place that has the most heaviness, pain, or tension. To the best of your ability, open to the sensations with curiosity and a willingness to suspend analysis or judgment. Just keep providing simple, kind attention. Let any emotions come to the surface.

Do not label the emotion but instead feel the raw sensation with openness. Observe when sensations shift. Do they soften? Is your attention drawn somewhere else in the body? Bring the same openness to that area. Do the sensations get more intense? Even if this feels uncomfortable, keep in mind that discomfort is part of the healing process.

Deepen your relationship with your body by opening to all of its ways of communicating. Pay attention to the emotions, images, information, and words that come to you. Finally, notice that amid the ever-changing emotions, sensations, and thoughts, there is a quiet presence that contains it all. Rest there, breathe, and be.

students to meditate with open but slightly downcast and relaxed eyes; if that feels comfortable to you, feel free to keep your eyes slightly open.

Allow Your Belly to Soften

One of the areas of chronic holding and blocked energy in the body is the lower abdomen. This is where people tend to protect their perceived vulnerability. Simply bringing your kind awareness to this area is enough to encourage the energy to release. For many practitioners, this deeply imbedded holding pattern returns over and again. But rest assured that in time after we've softened a thousand times, the pattern shifts.

Allow Your Breath to Deepen

In a meditation practice, it's essential to let go of controlling the breath in any way. You may find it helpful to take some deep breaths or do some yoga *pranayam* (breathing exercises) at the beginning of your meditation sitting, but make no effort to control your breath for most of your session. Once you soften the belly, you'll likely notice that your breath begins to deepen naturally. You may also notice some restriction or shallowness in your breathing. Or you may find that your breath speeds up in meditation. At these times, bring a gentle curiosity to the breath as it is. Notice that when you let go of control, the breath changes, softens, and becomes fuller on its own.

Bring Your Attention to Your Breath

The mind is used to having most of our attention most of the time. That's why most meditation styles give practitioners an alternative focus, such as a candle, hand movements, a mandala, a mantra, or a picture. This deep-healing meditation uses the breath as its focus. The breath works well because it's always available to us. If you find it too intense to feel the breath in the abdomen and chest, keep your attention near your nose, where the breath is more subtle. As your mind becomes less dominant, your body will relax. You may then feel it easier to shift your attention to the rhythm and sensations of the breath in the chest and belly.

Notice Other Sensations in Your Body

Open to other sensations in the body, starting with the pressure of your buttocks on your seat or the feel of your clothes brushing your skin. Notice these feelings with curiosity and let go of the need to adjust anything. You'll slowly find yourself becoming aware of more and more subtle sensations, including energy movements, pulsations, and tingling. Now is a good time to scan the chakras (chapter 2, page 17). Start with the heart and gradually move your focus upward to the throat, brow, and crown chakras. Then go back to the heart and gradually move your focus downward to the solar plexus, sacral, and root chakras. Spend thirty seconds to one minute in each chakra; or, if you feel inclined, spend more time. Notice images, impressions, insights, and sensations. Allow everything to be as it is.

Be Aware of Comfortable and Uncomfortable Sensations

It's imperative to begin to see everything as it is without classifying the experience as good or bad, desirable or undesirable. Take all sensations—such as comfort and discomfort, pleasure and displeasure—with equanimity. This attitude is the key to healing the physical body. Sensations are the primary way in which the soul communicates with you through the body, and in order to enter into an intimate relationship with the body and soul, you need to be open to hearing what's being said. If you're willing to listen and be open to whatever honestly arises, the relationship will mature. Like so many people, you may have been taught to disregard the body's messages for most of your life, and body-centered meditation begins the process of repairing the communication channels. When you're willing to open these channels, you receive many gifts, including physical healing, greater intuition, and deeper connection to the soul.

Think of a Health Condition You Want to Heal

When you call to mind a health challenge, you may feel physical discomfort, tension, and even energetic stagnation. You may not detect these sensations in the parts of the body related to your specific health concern, however, so remain open to the whole body. Bring your awareness to the area that seems to be asking for the most attention. You're likely to feel an emotion, one that you might call anger, fear, or sadness. Let go of labeling the emotion and instead simply be curious about the sensation. Keep an attitude of curiosity and openness and a willingness to let go of any concerns about what's being felt. Curious acceptance involves asking questions. Where do you feel the sensation? How big is it? Is it on the surface or is it deep? Is it moving or staying in the same place? Is there a temperature associated with it? A shape, texture, or color? Do any images, words, or memories appear? If so, let these come and go.

Be Aware of Heaviness, Pain, or Tension

The areas of your body that hold tension and discomfort are areas of blocked energy. Simple awareness is a powerful solvent of blocked energy. In other words, bringing acceptance and presence to these places sets the energy patterns free. My teacher, Adyashanti, has called this type of awareness "affectionate attention." Trying to control the energy, or even trying to help by manipulating it, often only serves to embed the patterns more deeply. This is because many of these attempts come from fear and trying to avoid what is.

Let Any Emotions Come to the Surface

As you practice over time, body-centered meditation will reveal many layers of blocked emotion. There's no avoiding these emotions, and they may be unpleasant at times. But remember that all emotions exist for good reasons and are in fact doorways into deep healing. You must allow the feelings and emotions to be as they are, and in the process, let them dance their way through and out of your system in their own time. As the layers of blocked emotions are released, more and more of your true nature will be revealed.

Observe When Sensations Shift

Often as a sensation softens in one part of the body, the energy flow picks up and affects other areas of the body. Consider this analogy: The energy body is like a city with many roads and highways. When one road is blocked, particularly a major road, it can affect the whole city. When congestion clears in one area, the traffic flow increases everywhere else. In the case of the energy system, the chakras are connected by a central channel called the *sushumna*. In addition, many smaller channels, or *nadi*, connect the rest of the energy body. For example, if you're feeling tightness in your chest and bring your awareness to it, your chest will soften and release blocked energy. You may then begin to feel tightness in your throat, which is not used to such an increase in energy flow. The increased energy flow is likely to pick up energy debris, or emotions anchored by false beliefs, in the newly opened channels. This is very positive but may temporarily feel uncomfortable; the discomfort will pass in its own time if you allow it.

Welcome Discomfort as Part of the Healing Process

When energetic sensations feel overwhelming, it's useful to remind yourself that energy is intelligent beyond your understanding and is always looking after your best and highest interest. Any sensation or emotion that's on the surface must be seen and allowed to move through. Discomfort as well as comfort have a place. Symptoms and disease have a place. Contemplate what this might mean for you. Let go of the battle against disease and symptoms. Instead, be still and listen. You'll find that when it comes to the body, there is no battle and never was one. The body is doing its very best given the current circumstances. Your job is to ask how you can help.

Deepen Your Relationship with Your Body

It takes great humility to just be open and listen, and the result can be very rewarding. Deep listening is a necessary step toward insight and healing. Deep listening may not give you instant answers, but it will give you true answers. Amid the ever-changing emotions, sensations, and thoughts, there's a quiet presence that contains it all.

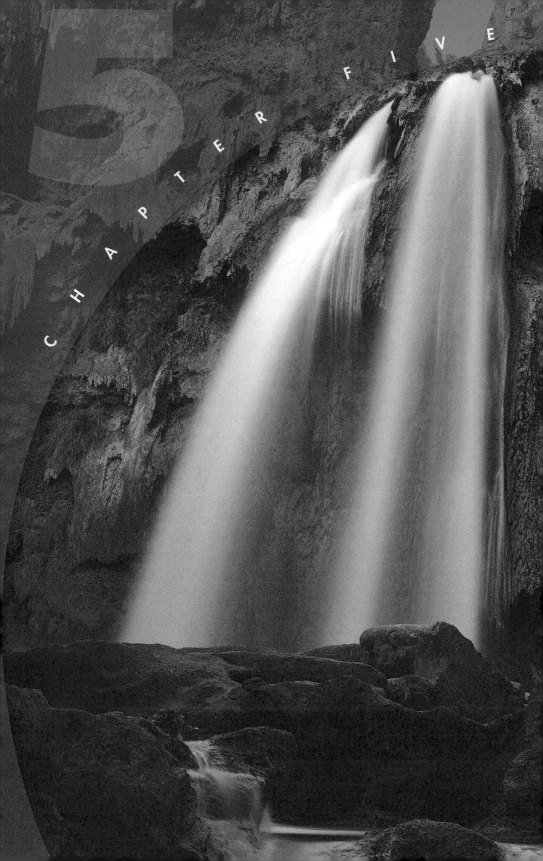

CHAPTER FIVE

Detoxification and Elimination

I wake sweet joy in dens of sorrow and I plant a smile
in forests of affliction, and wake the bubbling springs of life
in regions of dark death.

WILLIAM BLAKE

As we begin to adopt the deep-healing practices that we explored in the previous chapters, we support our growth in many ways. As we broaden our definition of health, we begin to see how our thoughts and emotions affect our choices and physical well-being. As we begin to dismantle our conditioning, we uncover a guidance system that unfailingly informs our perspective and directs us toward a new way of life. We recognize that all life is interconnected, and that beauty, happiness, health, and truth are available to us all. As blocked energy begins to flow, we once again begin to feel alive, creative, and inspired.

This chapter explores the process of detoxification: what it is, why it's needed, how it contributes to deep healing, and how it relates to our authentic growth. While most people think of detoxification, or cleansing, as a physical occurrence, it's really much more. During detoxification, we also encounter the many layers of emotions, false beliefs, and resistance that make up our own conditioning as well as the collective conditioning of society. In fact, we're all subject to an ongoing detoxification of beliefs, emotions, and energies that no longer serve us. This process is called retracing.

All deep-healing practices, including meditation, a plant-based diet, and regular juice fasts, can support retracing. These healing activities help us to detoxify because they revitalize our energy fields, bringing emotional fluidity, mental clarity, physical vigor, and spiritual connection.

TOXINS AND THEIR SOURCE

We wouldn't have to go through detoxification if we weren't subject to the many toxins that can originate outside or inside the body. Toxins that come from outside the body, which are also called exogenous toxins, enter through the mouth via food, prescription drugs, and water; through the skin via bathing water, cleaning products, and immunizations; and through the lungs via the air we breathe. These toxins, which include chemicals and heavy metals, have different origins. One common source is processed food, which contains chemicals that are added for flavor and texture, preservatives, refined fats and oils, sugar, and white flour. Other common sources of toxins include alcohol, amalgam dental fillings, cigarettes, cosmetics, household cleaners, industrial and urban pollution, off-gases from housing materials and furnishings, pesticides, plastics, radiation, and tap water. Exogenous toxins also come to us in the form of noise pollution and information overload from books, the Internet, newspapers, radio, and television.

Toxins that are produced inside the body, or endogenous toxins, include by-products of digestion, cellular wastes, fungal and parasite waste products, internally generated negative thoughts and emotions, putrefying food residues, and toxic chemical reactions. In addition, the body creates acidity if we consume excessive amounts of acid-forming foods, including processed foods, animal-based foods, and alcohol, and even too many acid-forming whole foods like grains, legumes, nuts, and seeds. Only vegetables and fruit are alkaline forming and they should ideally make up about three-quarters of the diet.

When we recognize the source of most toxins, we can make changes that allow us to avoid them. For example, we can choose nontoxic building materials, cleaning products, cosmetics, food and drink, and skin care products. In addition, we can install water purification systems and shower filters. Instead of using prescription drugs, we can opt to treat physical imbalances with acupuncture, food, herbs, homeopathy, and many other approaches that honor and support the body. We can lovingly free our lives of toxic people. Also, we can turn to spiritual practices, teachers, and therapists when we need help releasing false beliefs and stressful emotions.

When we're exposed to fewer toxins, our bodies gain vitality and we can begin the work of removing old, embedded toxins. As this process unfolds, we can expect emotional fluidity, enhanced intuition, inspired creativity, mental clarity, and a sense of inner peace and overall well-being. Physical changes include more energy, strong immunity, and improvements in processes such as digestion, elimination, menstruation, and sleep.

It's interesting to note that the more we connect with our authentic nature, the more we naturally avoid toxins and effortlessly make choices that support energy, health, and purity. We're less inclined to overconsume in general and also tend not to purchase products that are associated in any way with animal, human, or planetary suffering. As consumers we begin to live the awareness that everything is indeed connected.

FOOD CHOICES AND PHYSIOLOGICAL PROCESSES

The foods that we eat greatly influence detoxification and elimination. The body processes food in six distinct phases: intake, digestion, distribution, utilization, detoxification, and elimination. If we can minimize the time and energy spent on intake, digestion, distribution, and utilization, the body is able to mobilize more of its efforts toward detoxification and elimination. That's why a whole-foods, plant-based diet is the ideal deep healing diet (see chapter 8). This style of eating is easy on the digestive system, provides all the nutrients we need to thrive, leaves very few residual toxins for the body to deal with, and provides plenty of fiber to aid in elimination.

The human body has several routes of elimination, and these are used on a daily basis to excrete toxic substances that we've taken in through the lungs, mouth, and skin. In the deep healing process, it's essential that we eliminate substances that no longer serve us (or have never served us) or that have built up over time.

Five body systems are involved in elimination. Each system is composed of multiple organs and tissues. In addition, these systems and some organs are associated with specific spiritual lessons (see sidebar, page 31).

The Gastrointestinal System

The gastrointestinal system breaks down food into nutrients and wastes. It includes the colon, gallbladder, liver, and small intestine. Recommendations for supporting the colon and small intestine follow:

- Avoid foods that cause constipation, such as animal-based foods, crackers, dried fruits, and flour products.
- Eat a high-fiber, whole-foods diet that includes plenty of fruits and vegetables that have a high water content.
- Eat foods that enhance gut flora, such as cultured vegetables, kefir, miso, and yogurt. Also include chlorophyll-rich foods, such as chlorella, dark leafy greens, spirulina, sprouts, and wheatgrass products.

- Eat foods that lubricate the intestines, including alfalfa sprouts, almonds, apples, apricots, bananas, beets, carrots, cauliflower, honey, okra, peaches, pears, pine nuts, prunes, sea vegetables, sesame seeds, soy products, spinach, and walnuts.

- Eat foods that promote bowel movements, including asparagus, black sesame seeds, cabbage, coconut, figs, papaya, peas, sweet potatoes, and whole grains.

- Use enemas or colonics, particularly during a juice fast (see page 51 for more information).

- Use probiotics.

The liver and gallbladder area also part of the gastrointestinal system. Recommendations for supporting the gallbladder and liver follow:

- Avoid or eliminate alcohol.

- Decrease your overall food intake (unless you're malnourished).

- Eat foods that nourish the gallbladder and liver, including celery, cucumbers, green vegetables, legumes, millet, mung beans, radishes, tofu, and whole grains.

- Eat foods that rejuvenate the liver, including barley grass, chlorella, spirulina, wheatgrass products, and other green foods.

- Eat foods that stimulate the gallbladder and liver, including allium vegetables (members of the onion family), beets, broccoli, cabbage, cauliflower, cherries, cider vinegar, dandelion and other bitter leafy greens, peaches, strawberries, turnips, and raw foods in general.

- Eat the highest-quality food possible and make 75 percent of your diet fruits and vegetables.

- Eliminate processed fats and decrease your intake of other fats.

The Lymphatic System and the Skin

The lymphatic system filters bacteria and other particles out of body tissues and includes the lymph channels and lymph nodes. The body also releases toxins through the skin, sebaceous and sweat glands, and tears. Recommendations for supporting the lymphatic system and skin follow:

- Add ½ to 2 cups of epsom salts or sea salts to your bath and rinse well after bathing.

- Allow yourself to breathe deeply.

- Alternate cold and hot water when showering (see page 71 for more information).

- Expose yourself to gentle sunlight regularly.
- Engage in daily movement.
- Get a massage or bodywork.
- Take saunas and steam baths.
- Try dry brushing (see page 69 for more information).
- Use skin care products and cosmetics that contain only natural ingredients.

The Respiratory System

The respiratory system disposes of carbon dioxide. It includes the lungs and sinuses. Recommendations for supporting the respiratory system follow:

- Avoid mucus-forming foods, including dairy products, eggs, excessive grains, legumes, meat, nuts, poultry, and wheat.
- Avoid using chemical cleaners in the home.
- Engage in daily movement.
- Keep plants indoors and grow plants and trees outdoors.
- Sleep with the window slightly open, or sleep outdoors.
- Spend time in nature.
- Take saunas and steam baths.
- Use a neti pot regularly (see page 72 for more information).

The Urinary System

The urinary system involves the formation and release of urine. It includes the bladder, kidneys, and urethra. Recommendations for supporting the urinary system follow:

- Avoid intoxicants, such as alcohol, coffee, recreational drugs, and tobacco.
- Decrease or eliminate processed foods, poor-quality fats, and salt and salty condiments. Also decrease or eliminate high-protein foods, including animal-based foods, such as dairy products, eggs, and meat.
- Drink the purest water available.
- Eat foods that support the kidneys, including asparagus, beans, berries, celery, leafy greens, millet, oats, potatoes, quinoa, sea vegetables, gently cooked vegetables, and watermelon.
- Keep the area around your kidneys and lower back warm.

Spiritual Lessons

There are spiritual lessons associated with different body systems and organs. If you're having health challenges related to detoxification or elimination, what might your body be trying to tell you? Some examples follow:

BLADDER: Let go of fear-based emotions. What makes you anxious, fearful, or annoyed? How much of your fear is real and how much of it is imagined?

COLON: Learn from the past and let it go. Are you holding on to something (or someone) that is no longer serving you?

GALLBLADDER: Let go of bitterness and the past. What good has come from your past painful experiences?

KIDNEYS: Process fear and other stressful emotions. What do you give your power away to? How can you enhance your belief in yourself?

LIVER: Process and express anger in healthy ways. Do you need to set better boundaries and standards in relationships?

LUNGS: Breathe life in and allow yourself to be inspired. What choices do you make that impede your freedom?

LYMPHATIC SYSTEM: Allow yourself to be fully alive and present. Do you purposefully make yourself less noticeable? How can you show up more fully?

SINUSES: Enjoy and accept life as it is. Which parts of your life, including people and circumstances, do you resist?

SKIN: Feel safe being authentic. How do you doubt yourself? What does it feel like to just be yourself?

SMALL INTESTINE: Take in, absorb, and assimilate various aspects of your life. Are you exposing yourself to environments, people, or situations that are inappropriate for you?

THE HEALING CRISIS

At first, when you make the positive changes recommended for deep healing, you experience an increased feeling of well-being. This is always followed by a healing crisis, which can occur days, weeks, or even months later.

A healing crisis is not really a crisis. Rather, it's a sign of healing that can be subtle or quite obvious. It occurs when the body temporarily goes out of balance in order to find deeper balance and better health. A healing crisis is the body's way of excreting old toxins, both physical and emotional. In other words, as the body rebuilds, rests, and strengthens, it has the energy to heal more and more deeply.

You can recognize a healing crisis because it generally lasts for a few hours or up to one week and follows a period of improved food choices, increased self-care, or the beginning of a new holistic therapy. It often comes when you've been feeling better than ever, or when you're aware of an emotional component that has surfaced simultaneously with physical symptoms. Common symptoms include body aches, a coated tongue, diarrhea, fever, headache, or skin eruptions, and you might experience these without feeling sick or tired. Your particular symptoms are likely to mimic issues that you've had in the past. Even though you feel unwell physically and challenged emotionally, you're likely to have a deep, reassuring conviction that everything is okay during a healing crisis.

Although a healing crisis doesn't always involve being tired, it is possible that you experience temporary, deep weariness that feels different than physical fatigue. My sense is that this deep weariness is an energetic fatigue. When the body is on the edge of releasing old energies, we may become conscious of how tired we are of maintaining them. In fact, energetic weariness is often accompanied by the thought or words, "I just can't do this anymore. I'm so tired of this!"

If the popularity of caffeine, stimulants, and sugar is any indication, many people have an aversion to fatigue. However, it's crucial to let yourself experience it fully in order to let it go and make room for a new, more authentic, and empowered energy to emerge.

TRUST AND DEEP HEALING

The body is infinitely wise, and every body operates within a mystery that cannot be defined or predicted. In the end, every body heals in its own time and its own way. Rather than controlling the process, your energy is best spent on caring for your body and surrendering to the mystery of its healing.

Learning to trust the body is the greatest challenge we face, as many of us have been taught from childhood that the body is unreliable. On the whole, people in most developed societies have forgotten what it is to be a good steward of a physical body. Before we start school, most of us have been given antibiotics, drugs, and multiple vaccinations. Our fevers have been suppressed with aspirin, and our runny noses and coughs have been dried up with chemicals. We have been allowed

The Process

Many astute health practitioners have noticed that the body heals from the inside out. This means, for example, that the gallbladder will heal before a skin condition. The body also tends to heal from the top down, so the sinuses are likely to clear up before a foot fungus. Finally, recent symptoms heal before long-standing issues. So if you recently developed arthritis, the arthritis is likely to heal before the asthma you've had since childhood.

and even encouraged to eat foods on a daily basis that have little or no nutritional value. And before we reach our teens, many of us have experienced surgery and have routinely used prescription drugs to treat conditions such as asthma, attention deficit disorder, depression, and diabetes. From an early age, we're shown that the body is out of control and unintelligent.

Ultimately, trust in the body's ability to heal is innate and will be uncovered at some point during your deprogramming. Physical and spiritual wholeness follow naturally when you give the body and soul what they need to thrive.

DISEASE AND DEEP HEALING

*I*f you've been diagnosed with a disease, consider that any disease is simply a label that has been given to a set of symptoms that the body manifests when it's out of balance. It has taken many years for this disease to develop, and it will take time and effort to heal. When you adopt the principles of deep healing, you'll feel some positive changes almost instantly, whereas others may take months or even years.

The greatest challenge inherent in deep healing may be the collective fear that surrounds physical disease in general. Collective fear is an energy that we hold as a culture around death, which then manifests when we're "diagnosed" and given a label that says our body seems to be failing. But of course that belief is all wrong—if anything, we've failed the body by disregarding its sacred role in the marriage of soul and flesh.

Some labels trigger more fear than others. We need great courage to avoid getting caught up in the fear. We also need courage to clearly see that we're not living our own truth. Spirit is the only force that can supply the needed courage and spark the compassion and insight that are also necessary for transformation.

Along with the fear, we often feel anger toward the body because it won't do what we want it to. We must allow ourselves to feel the emotions that come up around our symptoms or disease; they are part of the energetic complex that has led to the symptoms. As the emotions are released, all of the energy that we've been using to suppress them can be freed up to help us access our intuition and heal deeply. Simultaneously, we show others the way and become energetic symbols of deep healing for our families and the larger community. Isn't that beautiful?

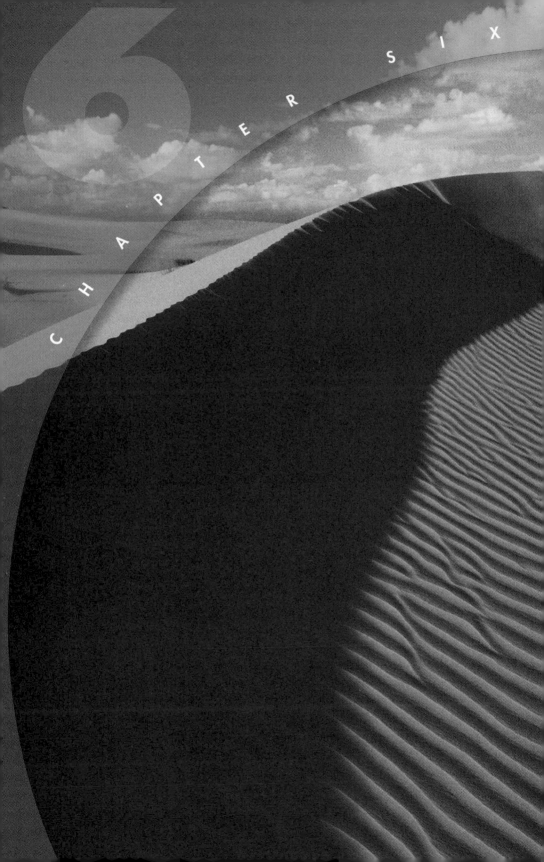

The Seven-Day Juice Fast

Fasting, in a larger context, means to abstain from that which is toxic to the mind, body, and soul. A way to understand this is that fasting is the elimination of physical, emotional, and mental toxins from our organism, rather than simply cutting down on or stopping food intake.

GABRIEL COUSENS, *SPIRITUAL NUTRITION AND THE RAINBOW DIET*

There are two primary nutritional causes for disease: an excess of accumulated toxins and a deficit of the nutrients the body needs to function optimally. The juice fast is a sound remedy that both cleanses and nourishes. In this chapter, I'll guide you through the deep-healing seven-day juice fast, which features freshly pressed juices, mineral broths, and tea infusions. The juice fast nourishes, strengthens, and regenerates your whole being.

Because this healthful liquid diet provides nutrients in a highly absorbable and concentrated form, very little effort will be required of your digestive system during the juice fast. Consequently, much of your energy will be freed up for detoxification and elimination, including the removal of deeply embedded toxins. The juice fast also gives glands, muscles, nerves, and other tissues a rest. In addition, fasting encourages the breakdown of diseased tissue, including abnormal cells, arterial plaque, gallstones, growths, kidney stones, and tumors.

Beyond purifying your body, the juice fast helps clear your mind and free stuck emotional energy. This is important because tissues contract around old emotions that are being held in the body, which hinders cleansing and nourishing and creates the opportunity for disease to take hold.

Meditating during the juice fast can create the ideal environment for clearing stagnant emotions and energies. Where there is an inner stillness, there is a freeing of blocked energy. When energy is released, there is relaxation and an opening of both the energy body and the physical body. This leads to spiritual and physical nourishment, as well as the release of emotional and physical debris. For a sample deep-healing meditation, see page 36.

PREPARING FOR THE JUICE FAST

*W*hile juice fasts are generally safe and helpful for everyone, you should seek the counsel of a holistic health practitioner who is knowledgeable about fasting if you have concerns. It's a particularly good idea to consult an expert if you've had difficulties fasting in the past, have a medical condition, or are taking prescription drugs.

Besides reading this chapter to prepare for the deep-healing seven-day juice fast, the most important step you can take before beginning is to clarify your intention. Why do you want to do the fast? The deeper your reasons for undertaking the fast, the more committed and engaged you will be once you begin.

I lead community juice fasts that give participants the opportunity to go through the fasting experience together. At the beginning of each fast, I suggest that they write down why they want to do the fast. We put the intentions in an envelope, seal it, and burn it on the last day of the fast. The envelope sits on my altar at home throughout the fast. Completing the same simple exercise can help you clarify your intentions for fasting too. Write down the following:

- three things you would like to welcome into your life
- three things you would like to let go of
- the name of someone you would like to dedicate your fast to, such as someone who is sick or has greatly influenced you

When to Fast

It's possible to fast and continue your regular activities, but it can be helpful to take the full week, or at least a few days, away from your regular responsibilities so you can focus on deep healing. Although it's important to find an opportune time in your schedule, keep in mind that the optimal times to fast are when you're feeling unwell, your digestion is compromised, you don't find food appealing, or your intuition says its time. In addition, you might want to plan the fast for a time when you can do it with others, such as during a community juice fast.

Twice each year, I hold community juice fasts and invite my clients to participate. I do this because I believe that when people gather with the shared intention of nurturing their bodies and souls, they create a

Fast Alternative: the Week-long Cleanse

If you're not ready to do the juice fast just yet, you can still add freshly pressed juices, mineral broths, and tea infusions to your diet. In fact, instead of doing a seven-day juice fast, you could do a week-long cleanse that includes juice, mineral broths, and tea infusions along with fruits, green smoothies, salads, and raw and steamed vegetables. A typical day might start with a tea infusion, followed by a green smoothie, then a big salad at lunch, with a juice and some fruit in the afternoon and plenty of steamed vegetables or a vegetable soup in the evening. Just as you would during a fast, include some of the cleansing practices described in chapter 7.

strong energy current that can dissolve common cultural beliefs—and their corresponding emotions—about the body and disease. The group environment is fun and supportive, and participants feel more confident, informed, prepared, and relaxed.

Enjoy your fast in silence if that's possible. Turn off the cell phone, computer, radio, and television. If you can't do this at home, consider your options for a peaceful getaway, perhaps to a cottage by the water or a place in the country.

If you can fast when you have few responsibilities, you're likely to experience a deep unwinding that's precious beyond words. You can wake up when you want, nap as often as you need to, spend as much time on additional cleansing practices (see chapter 7) as you'd like, take long walks, write in a journal, and meditate.

Don't skip the juice fast simply because you never seem to have the time. Keep in mind that clearing most obligations aside from your regular work schedule can be a suitable compromise. For example, if you're a weekday nine-to-fiver, reserve your evenings and weekends. Plan to make mineral broths and tea infusions in advance and transport them to work in thermoses. Just before leaving for work, make a big batch of fresh juice to take with you. Just be sure to keep the juice cold to prevent oxidation.

One Week Before the Fast

Plan to make certain preparations during the week before your fast. For example, ask for your family's support. Tell them why the fast is important to you and let them know you'll need time to yourself during the fast. If you usually cook for the family, plan accordingly. Possible strategies include preparing and freezing meals in advance and asking the family to make some of their own meals that week. If you can schedule times for the children to visit friends or grandparents, you won't need to

The Juice Fast Shopping List

Following is a suggested shopping list that includes the produce you'll need for freshly pressed juice for one person for three to four days. Of course, your needs may vary based on your preferences. Before shopping, also refer to the recipes for Mineral Broth (page 96) and the tea infusions (pages 87 to 95) to add the necessary ingredients to your shopping list.

FOR THE JUICE:

Fruits

ginger, 1 (4- to 6-inch) root	lemons, 10	oranges, 5 pounds
grapefruits, 4	limes, 3	pineapple, 1
green apples, 5 pounds		

Vegetables

beets, 3 pounds	fennel bulb, 1	red bell peppers, 2
cabbage, 1 head	green onions, 1 bunch	romaine lettuce, 1 to 2 heads
carrots, 5 to 10 pounds	kale, 2 bunches	spinach, 2 bunches
celery, 3 heads	parsley, 1 to 2 bunches	tomatoes, 5
cucumbers, 4		

worry about meals during those times. Plus, you'll have more time alone to concentrate on your own needs.

Another important step is to change your diet this week. Have fresh-pressed juice at least once each day. Try to have a green smoothie and a salad every day too. This is a gentle way of preparing yourself for the seven-day juice fast. Following are some daily guidelines that might be helpful:

- six to seven days prior: avoid all processed foods
- five to six days prior: avoid all animal-based foods
- three to four days prior: avoid all flour products and decrease oils and nut butters
- two to three days prior: decrease nuts and seeds
- one to two days prior: eat only fruits, legumes, sprouts, and fresh raw and steamed vegetables; use cold-pressed oils sparingly

One additional step is to wean yourself off of stimulants and supplements, which you won't be using during the fast. Gradually decrease your consumption of coffee and other caffeinated drinks. Also, stop taking vitamin and mineral supplements before starting the fast.

The Juice Fast: a Typical Day

During the juice fast, your priority is to listen to your body. Have your juice and other clear drinks when the time feels right for you. Your needs may change from day to day. However, here's an example of what a typical day might look like:

7 a.m.	tea infusion	2 p.m.	fresh juice
8 a.m.	wheatgrass shot	4 p.m.	tea infusion
10 a.m.	fresh juice	6 p.m.	fresh juice
noon	mineral broth		

During this week as well as the week of the fast, plan on going to bed as early as possible every evening. In addition, toward the end of the week, plan a big shopping trip to get the ingredients you need for the juice and mineral broth. See page 54 for a sample shopping list. Keep in mind that this list will keep you stocked for three to four days; plan a second shopping trip for additional fresh produce during the fast.

DURING THE FAST

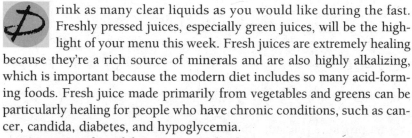

rink as many clear liquids as you would like during the fast. Freshly pressed juices, especially green juices, will be the highlight of your menu this week. Fresh juices are extremely healing because they're a rich source of minerals and are also highly alkalizing, which is important because the modern diet includes so many acid-forming foods. Fresh juice made primarily from vegetables and greens can be particularly healing for people who have chronic conditions, such as cancer, candida, diabetes, and hypoglycemia.

As a general guideline, you can drink up to two quarts (about two liters) of fresh juice each day of the fast. If you're drawn to sweeter juices, such as those made from apples, beets, carrots, and oranges, try to have these before or after exercise so that you quickly burn the sugars. The other clear liquids you can drink include mineral broths; tea infusions; wheatgrass juice; herbal teas, such as chaga tea; purified water; and fresh coconut water. More information about these beverages follows; for specific recipes, see pages 87 to 97.

Freshly Pressed Juices

During the fast, plan to make fresh juice twice each day by putting lots of fresh vegetables and some fruit through a juicer to remove the fiber. Do

How to Choose a Juicer

There are many types of juicers on the market today. Generally, a single or twin gear masticating juicer is best. Masticating juicers are relatively easy to clean and effectively juice vegetables, including leafy greens, as well as fruit. Twin gear juicers, such as Green Power and Green Star, produce excellent juice. They also tend to be a little more expensive, have bigger motors, and take up more counter space. There are also vertical single gear juicers, such as Hurom and Omega, that take up less counter space and are efficient, quiet, and self-feeding. When selecting a juicer, choose one that has a slow rotation speed so that the fruits and vegetables aren't exposed to heat and denatured as they're being juiced.

If you're new to juicing or are simply on a tight budget, you might want to ask friends and family if you can borrow a juicer while you decide if you want to purchase your own. You can also try purchasing a secondhand juicer online.

not use commercial juices that come in bottles, cans, or cartons during the fast. The vast majority of juices sold in stores are pasteurized, which destroys nutrients. However, if you live near a fresh juice bar, you may find it helpful, and a welcome treat, to purchase some juices there.

It takes quite a large amount of vegetables and fruit to produce one eight-ounce glass of juice, making freshly pressed juice one of the most concentrated sources of nutrients available. Your digestive system—specifically, the uppermost part of the small intestine—is able to access all of this glorious nutrition in minutes. Studies have shown that juicing foods does not significantly decrease nutrient levels, especially if the juice is consumed right after preparation. For convenience during the fast, you may want to make a large quantity of fresh juice at once. This is okay provided you store the fresh juice in a sealed container in the refrigerator and drink it within a few hours of making it. Your taste buds will tell you how fresh the juice is.

When you're not fasting, fresh juices can be a supplement to your regular meals. You can drink juice between meals, or even right before meals, and still have room for solid food.

Mineral Broths

Many food sources today are deficient in minerals, and as a result, our bodies are too. The primary cause is the depleted condition of most soils, due to intensive farming practices. In the body, mineral stores are eroded when we consume refined foods, particularly sugar and white flour; eat acid-forming foods, such as animal-based foods and refined foods; fail to eat sufficient quantities of fruits and vegetables; and drink coffee and carbonated beverages.

Mineral broths are a simple and economical way to add minerals to your diet, and doing so will benefit every system in your body. In addition, making a mineral broth is a great way to use the inedible or leftover parts of vegetables, as well as vegetables that are past their prime. I keep a large container in the fridge and add vegetable trimmings to it as I prepare meals during the week. At the end of the week, I include these trimmings when making mineral broth. I like to drink the broth warm, use it as a base for soup, or use it in place of water when cooking grains.

I've included a recipe for mineral broth on page 96, but once you get the hang of making it, you'll no longer need to refer to a strict ingredient list. Simply use up what you have in the fridge and pantry. For example, use carrots and other root vegetables that are soft or shriveled; greens that are starting to become pale; onions and potatoes that have started to sprout; and any other vegetables, such as beets, cabbage, celery hearts, and squash, that you want to use up. For the best flavor, make sure that beets, carrots, potatoes, sweet potatoes, and squash make up at least half of the vegetables in each batch.

Mineral broths allow you to access all the nutrients from the bits of vegetables that aren't typically used. For example, use leftover asparagus ends; broccoli, cauliflower, collard green, kale, and mushroom stems; cabbage cores; carrot and celery leaves; corn silk; and dark leek greens.

Another healthful ingredient for mineral broth is sea vegetables, which are an excellent source of highly concentrated bulk and trace minerals, including iodine. Use arame, dulse, kelp, kombu, and nori. Be aware: a small amount of flavorful sea vegetables goes a long way.

Finally, if you have access to wild greens, they're a wonderful addition to mineral broth. For example, use dandelion greens, garlic mustard greens, mallow, nettles, purslane, and wild spinach.

Tea Infusions

Tea infusions are concentrated preparations made from nutritious and healing herbs that alkalize, balance, and rebuild the body. In this way, they differ from cleansing teas, which stimulate detoxification. In addition, tea infusions are stronger than most teas because they're made from a much greater amount of herbs and they steep longer.

I like to use locally grown dried herbs when making tea infusions, but an alternative is to purchase dried herbs in bulk from a natural food store or online supplier. You can make your infusions from a single herb or try combining them, as is done for Nourishing Tea Infusion (page 87). Tea infusions provide the most benefit when used regularly.

When making tea infusions, I choose herbs that are beneficial for the entire system and are safe for the whole family. Following is information about some of my favorite herbs and their healing properties:

NETTLE LEAVES. Valuable for the whole system, nettle leaves nourish and strengthen the circulatory system; digestive system; endocrine glands, including the ovaries and testes; kidneys; lungs; and nervous system. A great source of iron, nettle leaves also promote joint health and stabilize blood sugar.

OAT STRAW. An excellent source of calcium, oat straw strengthens the bones, hair, nails, and teeth. It promotes deep sleep and relaxation, nourishes the nervous system, decreases cholesterol levels, strengthens the liver, and stabilizes blood sugar levels.

RASPBERRY LEAVES. Rich in minerals, raspberry leaves generally strengthen the whole system, particularly the reproductive system. Raspberry leaves also help to build the blood, bones, teeth, and tissues.

RED CLOVER BLOSSOMS. Both nourishing and alkalizing, red clover blossoms purify the blood, which supports healthy growth and fights cancerous growth. Red clover blossoms also balance the endocrine system and liver, ease inflammation, and promote healthy skin and joints.

Wheatgrass Juice

Wheatgrass juice and the juice of other young grasses, such as barley and oats, can be a valuable addition to your juice-fasting regimen. One option is to buy fresh wheatgrass juice at a nearby juice bar. If that's not feasible, you can explore a few other alternatives. The simplest option is to purchase frozen wheatgrass juice, which is available at most natural food stores or can be ordered online. Another option is to purchase fully grown wheatgrass at a natural food store or farmers' market and run it through your juicer. The final but more challenging alternative is to grow wheatgrass yourself. While this choice gives you the freshest wheatgrass and the most control over quality, it also takes time and planning.

Wheatgrass juice is valued for its alkalizing and anti-inflammatory properties; in addition, it boasts a high concentration of chlorophyll, which makes it a powerful blood builder and detoxifier. Wheatgrass juice also contains a broad spectrum of amino acids, antioxidants, enzymes, essential fatty acids, vitamins, and minerals. In fact, wheatgrass can contain more than ninety minerals, which are essential for rebuilding the body. Wheatgrass also contains an unnamed component, sometimes referred to as the "grass juice factor," which supports deep healing and cellular regeneration. This effect may be attributed in part to an enzyme called P4D1 that stimulates the renewal of RNA and DNA, the key components in cell duplication. Overall, the high concentration of enzymes in wheatgrass juice helps to break down diseased tissues in the body.

Wheatgrass juice is generally taken on its own in two-ounce "shots." If you incorporate wheatgrass juice into your juice fast, be sure to rotate its use with other juices. For most people, one or two shots per day can be a helpful addition to the juice fast. However, you can have up to five shots per day; greater quantities are especially appropriate if you've been diagnosed with a serious disease. For example, wheatgrass juice is commonly recommended for people who have cancer.

Purified Water

It's important to drink water that has been purified, which means that chemicals, including chlorine, and heavy metals have been filtered out. Many home filtration devices are available. I have a Santevia system in my kitchen and am quite happy with it. This type of system removes toxins and chlorine and also adds minerals, making the purified water alkaline and similar in composition to spring water. In addition, the water is restructured so that it's more absorbable.

Other Considerations

The juice fast is a potent time for not only physical renewal but also emotional healing, mental rest, and spiritual connection. To get the most benefit from the fast, limit entertainment and socializing and instead concentrate on inner stillness, self-care, and settling into natural time by letting your days unfold rather than rushing around.

Meditation and journaling are two practices that can help you accept the emotions that come up during the fast. Light exercise, such as walking and gentle yoga, are also good practices, in part because they help cleanse the lymphatic system. However, heavy training should be avoided, because you want to harness as much energy as possible for healing. For additional cleansing, consider seeing a trusted health practitioner for energy work or body work.

Chapter 7 features additional detoxifying techniques that you might want to incorporate into your fast. These practices, which originate from ancient and traditional approaches to holistic health, help the body access and remove accumulated toxins. You can continue these healthful practices as part of your regular routine after the fast.

BREAKING THE FAST

reaking the fast in a wise and gentle way is as important as the fast itself. Many people make the mistake of going back to their regular diet too quickly, which can tax the digestive system. The best strategy is to have a light menu for a few days before slowly easing back into your regular diet or transitioning to the everyday deep-healing diet (see chapter 8).

For three to four days following the fast, select plant-based foods, including raw and steamed vegetables, fruits, gluten-free grains, legumes, sprouts, nuts, and seeds. Juices, smoothies, and soups are excellent choices because they're easy on the digestive system.

Your bathroom habits are likely to change during the fast, but about two days after you break the fast, you should have a bowel movement. If not, try soaking a handful of prunes overnight and eating them along with the soak water the next morning.

Good Bacteria

It's important to add good bacteria back to your diet after the juice fast, especially if you've done enemas. Even if you haven't included enemas, it's wise to replenish gut microorganisms. These humble bacteria are essential for deep healing, and they're more necessary now than ever because antibiotics, chlorine, and processed foods tend to strip them out of our systems. Although a healthy digestive tract has three to four pounds of good bacteria, which resides mostly in the colon, the vast majority of people lack these beneficial bacteria.

Helpful gut flora has many functions, such as keeping the bowels clean and enhancing elimination; keeping fungus and parasites in check; neutralizing toxic substances; and producing vitamins, particularly the B vitamins. In fact, some experts believe that good bacteria are 80 percent responsible for the health of the immune system.

The best way to replenish good bacteria is by consuming fermented and unpasteurized foods, which is a common practice among traditional cultures. Foods such as kefir, kimchi, miso, sauerkraut, fermented vegetables, and yogurt have been used for generations. The vegetable-based foods are my preference, because many people now have difficulty digesting dairy products. However, some people who cannot consume dairy may be able to tolerate organic yogurt made from goat's or sheep's milk. In comparison with cows, these animals produce milk that is more similar to human milk. The proteins are smaller and easier to digest, making them less likely to cause physical disturbances.

Another, and quite expedient, option is to take probiotic supplements, which are available at any natural food store. However, as a

Breaking the Fast

As you break the fast, notice how you feel after you add new foods. Assess your emotions, energy level, and satisfaction with meals. If you feel discomfort or are feeling unwell, which may happen when you introduce heavier foods, go back to eating lighter fare for a day or two.

Following are some suggested items to include on your menu as you break the fast:

DAY ONE: fruit, green smoothies, sprouts, and raw vegetables

DAY TWO: add gluten-free grains, legumes, steamed vegetables, and cold-pressed oil

DAY THREE: add raw nuts and seeds

nutritionist, I consider fermented foods to be the more reliable and effective choice. For a sample fermented food recipe, see Basic Cultured Vegetables (page 118).

AFTER THE FAST

After completing the seven-day fast and breaking the fast appropriately, you have many opportunities to continue nourishing and cleansing throughout the year. For example, the period following a fast is the perfect time to adopt the everyday deep healing diet (see chapter 8). Another option is to simplify your diet one day each week by consuming only fresh juices or eating only fruits and vegetables. If it feels more manageable, an alternative is to make this diet shift from noon of one day to noon of the next day. In addition, consider doing this "mini-cleanse" for two to three days every quarter; particularly good times are when the seasons are changing.

The very last consideration after completing the fast is planning when you want to do it again. Remember, the benefits of deep healing continue and deepen with each fast. Every fast provides a new opportunity to address another level of physical and emotional health.

Juice Fast FAQs

Will I feel hungry?

Yes, you likely will feel hungry at times during the fast, although some people report not feeling hungry at all. But don't worry: Unless you're emaciated, you'll have more than enough reserves to make it through a week without solid foods. In addition, you'll be receiving plenty of nutrients, arguably more than you usually do. The juices, broths, and teas will deliver ample carbohydrates, fats, minerals, phytonutrients, proteins, and vitamins.

What can I do to cope with hunger?

When you feel hungry, soften to it. In other words, don't brace against it. Be open and curious about the sensations associated with hunger. Soften your jaw, belly, throat, shoulders, and forehead. Notice how hunger comes and goes, and how it abates when you haven't eaten anything at all. Finally, notice that when you're relaxed, hunger is less uncomfortable.

What if I cheat and fail?

Bring awareness to this concern and the sensations that accompany it. Realize that cheating and failure exist only in your mind. If you eat something solid, you can always resume the fast. There's no perfect juice fast. Like anything else, the fast provides an opportunity for both good and bad tendencies to reveal themselves. Food addictions and your inner critic are likely to show up. By being as mindful as you can be of the cravings, emotions, energies, and thoughts that arise, you can limit their influence.

Can I shorten the fast to a weekend?

Giving your body a break from digestion while nourishing it with juice, broths, and teas is always valuable. So yes, you can fast for one day, or two or three. However, the first couple days of a juice fast are usually the most challenging. By day three the system adjusts, and the experience can become quite pleasant. Some of my best physical experiences and spiritual epiphanies have occurred during the latter days of a juice fast.

Can I exercise during a fast?

It's best to avoid heavy exercise during a juice fast so your body can focus its energy on healing. Walks and gentle movement are fine for most people. However, I've guided fast participants who were training for endurance events and didn't want to depart from their training schedules. They were able to successfully combine the fast along with their exercise regimens. In addition, they found that consuming sweeter juices before or after training was helpful.

Will I lose weight on a fast?

Everyone loses weight on a juice fast, and most people are happy about that. If you're already at a comfortable weight, you'll regain what you lose within about two weeks of resuming your regular diet. Because it brings balance to the system, juice fasting helps you to settle at a healthy weight over time, as long as your regular diet and lifestyle are healthy. In addition, the emotional and spiritual healing that occurs during a juice fast helps support a balanced weight.

Will my metabolism shut down?

That is a possibility, but I feel it depends on the attitude you bring to the fast. The body goes into storage mode when it feels deprived. When you are very clear on why you're fasting, are willing to slow down, and focus on nourishing yourself spiritually so that emotional energy can be released, there is a freeing of the energy body which leads to a balanced metabolism, and of course heath-supportive choices when you go back to eating solid foods..

I tend to be cold most of the time. What can I do to keep myself warm during a juice fast?

In general, people feel cooler during a juice fast for two reasons. First, much of our body heat is generated by the digestion of solid foods. And second, most juice ingredients tend to be cooling. Your body should adapt over the course of the fast and generate more heat, particularly as your health improves and your adrenal glands recover. If you always tend to feel cool, your adrenal glands may be overworked, so let them rest. Don't fill up your schedule; instead, take time to unwind, both during the fast and always.

To keep warm, dress in layers and exercise in short bursts throughout the day to generate heat. In addition, drink warm broths and teas between juices.

When making juice, choose warming vegetables, such as cabbage, garlic, green onion, and ginger. Beets and carrots are neutral, so they're also good choices. Cooling vegetables include celery, cucumbers, leafy greens, and tomatoes. Combine them with warming vegetables. Fruit is generally cooling, although cherries are warming and grapes and pineapple are neutral. When making broths, include beets, cabbage, carrots, garlic, and onions.

Will I get enough protein?

Juices contain some protein, but of course they're lower in protein than our usual diets. When the body gets less protein through the diet, it begins to break down proteins in unhealthy cells, growths, and tumors. It also breaks down arterial plaque, gallstones, and kidney stones. This is one of the reasons why a fast is so healing. When we're not fasting, the system is rarely encouraged to do this kind of scavenging because most of us consume an excessive amount of protein.

How long do juices keep?

The ideal is to drink freshly made juice. At the same time, you don't want juicing to become an unpleasant chore. My suggestion is to drink freshly pressed juice within six hours. When I fast I juice twice a day, once in the morning and once in the afternoon. Each time I juice, I make enough for two eight-ounce glasses. I store any juice that I don't drink immediately in the refrigerator.

Juicing removes fiber, but isn't fiber important?

Temporarily removing fiber from your diet allows your digestive system to easily absorb nutrients without much effort so your small intestine can completely rest and focus its energy on excretion. When you return to eating solid foods, fiber is indeed important, and I encourage you to consume a high-fiber, whole-food diet in addition to fresh juices.

Can I fast longer than seven days?

If you sense that you're in the midst of an important process and are not quite ready to return to solid foods, by all means continue the fast. However, I recommend you seek guidance from an experienced health practitioner if the fast extends to more than three weeks. Many people have undertaken juice fasts that have lasted between forty and 100 days with no negative consequences; in fact, when done correctly, a long fast can result in many seemingly miraculous improvements.

Most important, make sure the desire to continue fasting comes from your soul and not your ego. When you make a decision from the soul, you'll feel a deep relaxation in the body.

Are water fasts more effective than juice fasts?

A water fast is extremely powerful because the body spends even less energy processing nutrients than it does during a juice fast, which frees even more resources for the process of detoxification. My concern is that many people lack minerals and other nutrients that are necessary for the body's functioning, and a water fast can potentially contribute to this depletion. The beauty of a juice fast is that it replenishes the body's reserves. However, if you've done multiple juice fasts and sense that your nutrient stores are healthy, you can add one or more water-only days to the juice fast and see how that feels for you.

Is it safe to fast if I have a disease?

If you're worried that the body will be overwhelmed, rest assured that it won't release more toxins than it can handle. Additional cleansing practices (see chapter 7) can help rid the body of toxins. I highly recommend enemas or colonics and castor oil packs for your liver, along with any other cleansing practices that appeal to you. If you don't feel ready to do a juice fast, however, try a week-long cleanse (see sidebar, page 53).

Can I drink one cup of fresh nut milk each day during the fast?

I would leave nut milks out of the cleanse because they contain more fat and protein, and the body will spend energy breaking down these fats and proteins instead of breaking down diseased tissue. However, if adding nut milks feels comforting for you, then feel free to do so.

Why am I awake in the middle of the night?

Some people report waking at night during a fast, while others sleep more soundly. To avoid waking, try not to drink anything close to bedtime. If you wake up at night, I suggest you bring your awareness to your breath and body and do a lying-down meditation, noticing the sensations in your body.

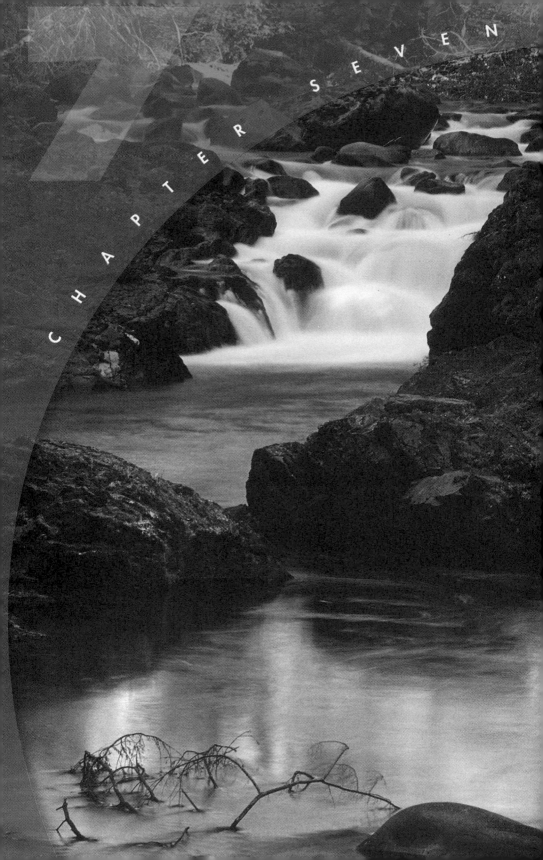

Additional Cleansing Practices

So just take whatever steps seem easiest for you, and as
you take a few steps it will become easier for you to take a
few more.

PEACE PILGRIM

In this chapter I list many practices that you can incorporate into the
seven-day juice fast. As you read, note which ones you're drawn to; the
attraction to certain practices is intuitive. Your body knows what it needs
right now. During subsequent fasts, you may feel comfortable adding more
practices as the first ones you try become familiar.

In addition to performing some of the following practices, try to get out in
the sun and fresh air every day during the fast. This is also a good time to take
saunas, soak in sea salt or Epsom salt baths, and use essential oils. If possible, promote detoxification by visiting your favorite body or energy worker.

Castor Oil Packs

Castor oil is a vegetable oil that should not be taken internally. A castor oil pack
is placed on the skin to increase circulation, promote elimination, and heal the
tissues and organs underneath the skin. Castor oil packs are used for many conditions, including arthritis; constipation; eczema; female reproductive imbalances;
gallbladder, kidney, and liver problems; psoriasis; and warts and other growths.

Castor oil has an extremely high content of ricinoleic acid, which prevents
the growth of bacteria, molds, viruses, and yeasts. It also increases lymphocyte
production and the activity level of T-cell lymphocytes that originate in the
bone marrow and thymus gland. These lymphocytes identify and kill invaders,
such as bacteria, cancer, fungi, and viruses. Castor oil strengthens the immune
system and increases the flow of lymph throughout the body, speeding the

DEEP HEALING

Suggested Morning Routine

When incorporating multiple practices into the juice fast, the most important consideration is choosing activities that you like and have time for. Following is a suggested morning regimen that includes many cleansing practices. This particular routine takes a couple of hours to complete. If you find you're rushing through it, adjust accordingly. You may not be able to do the full routine every morning, so shorten it when needed.

- Wake up naturally.
- Brush your teeth and scrape your tongue *(see page 73)*.
- Drink two mugs of tea infusion *(see page 87)* or two glasses of purified water.
- Use a neti pot *(see page 72)*.
- Try oil pulling *(see page 72)*.

- Have an enema *(see page 70)*.
- Dry brush your skin *(see opposite page)*.
- Shower using hot-and-cold water therapy *(see page 71)*.
- Drink wheatgrass juice *(see page 58)*.
- Meditate *(see chapter 4)*.
- Prepare and drink fresh juice *(see chapter 6)*.

removal of toxins from cells. It also appears to balance the autonomic nervous system, improve digestion, and increase liver activity.

During a fast and at other times, a castor oil pack can be placed over abnormal skin growths or skin conditions, areas affected by bursitis, inflamed and swollen joints, and muscle strains. A castor oil pack also can be placed on the right side of the abdomen to stimulate the liver, in the middle of the abdomen to relieve constipation and other digestive disorders, and on the lower abdomen to relieve menstrual irregularities and ovarian and uterine cysts. Castor oil should not be applied to broken skin or used during menstruation, pregnancy, or breastfeeding.

Some natural food stores and online retailers sell ready-made castor oil packs. It's also easy to make your own. Here's what you'll need:

- a piece of cotton or wool flannel large enough to cover the affected area when folded into two to four layers
- castor oil (try to find the Palma Christi brand, which is sold at many natural food stores)
- sheets of plastic wrap (another option is to use a plastic shopping bag; if the bag is printed, turn it inside-out so that the castor oil can't come into contact with the ink)
- a hot water bottle or heating pad
- old pajamas and towels or sheets (castor oil will stain clothing and bedding)

- a container with a lid (so you can store and reuse the pack)

To administer the castor oil pack, follow these general guidelines:

- Fold the flannel so that it is two to four layers thick and large enough to cover the affected area. Put the flannel on a sheet of plastic cut 1 to 2 inches larger than the folded flannel or simply use an inside-out plastic shopping bag. Pour castor oil onto the flannel until it is saturated but not dripping.

- Place an old towel or sheet on the bed where you'll be resting. Lie down.

- Flip the pack so that the soaked cloth is directly on the skin of the affected area with the plastic on top.

- Place the hot water bottle or heating pad (set on medium) over the pack. Leave it on for 40 to 60 minutes. Rest while the pack is in place, meditating and envisioning the affected areas functioning perfectly. Along with your vision, concentrate on the associated feelings of empowerment, gratitude, and trust. You could also play relaxing music and light a candle while you're using the pack.

- After removing the pack, cleanse the area with a dilute solution of water and baking soda if desired. To make the solution, stir 1 teaspoon of baking soda into 2 cups of water.

- Store the pack in a covered jar or plastic container in the refrigerator. Each pack may be reused 25 to 30 times if stored properly. Add a little fresh oil each time you use the pack, and use castor oil packs on alternating days rather than every day.

Dry Skin Brushing

The skin is the largest organ of elimination. It releases great amounts of body waste, but its function can be inhibited by dead skin cells, excreted toxins, external pollution, and skin care products. If your skin cannot efficiently release toxins, you may experience acne, body odor, eczema, hives, itchiness, rashes, and psoriasis. If toxins are unable to escape through the skin, they'll either be stored in fat cells, which contributes to cellulite and other fatty deposits, or they'll be recirculated back into the bloodstream, which overworks the kidneys, liver, and other organs. Dry skin brushing removes dead skin cells and stimulates the flow of lymph, the fluid that surrounds cells. It also increases blood flow to the skin and improves overall skin health.

Choose a dry skin brush that has natural fiber bristles and a long handle so you can reach your back. Follow these guidelines:

- Brush your dry body before you shower or bathe, preferably in the morning.
- Start at your feet and always brush toward your heart. Use long strokes on the legs, buttocks, abdomen, back, arms, and shoulders and circular motions on the joints. Use a figure eight motion around the breasts, avoiding the nipples. You might find yourself using a combination of circular and long movements on some areas of the body, which is fine. Just remember to brush in the general direction of the heart.
- Adjust the pressure according to the sensitivity of the skin and the area of the body.
- Avoid brushing anywhere the skin is broken or where you have a cut, infection, rash, or wound.
- Finish by taking a shower. If you choose, use hot-and-cold water therapy (see opposite page) to further stimulate the lymphatic system and improve circulation.
- Dry off vigorously and massage pure plant oils—such as almond, coconut, jojoba, or sesame oil—into your skin.

Enemas

The colon is the drain of the human body. When elimination is impeded, the whole system becomes backed up with metabolic waste. Over the course of your lifetime, debris from animal-based foods and refined foods accumulates on the walls of the colon. Over time, the debris forms into tar-like plaque that can prevent absorption and elimination, which creates an environment ripe for infection, inflammation, and abnormal growths, including cancer. Colon cancer is currently one of the most common forms of cancer.

A juice fast can be an ideal time to not only rest the colon but also help it to slough off accumulated plaque by using enemas. Because no fiber is being taken in during the fast, the colon will be empty of food after a couple of days. That's when an enema can work on removing debris from the colon walls. Most people are quite surprised to see how much fecal matter is still being eliminated even after one week of fasting and daily enemas. This fecal matter can range from silt-like liquid to rubbery stools to parasites. It may not be pleasant to read about such things, but I always say better out than in!

Once you start the juice fast, you'll likely have a bowel movement the morning of the first day and possibly the second day. Since there will be no more fiber in your system, you're unlikely to have a natural bowel movement after that. The best time to start the enemas is in the morning on the second day of the fast. It's safe to continue the enemas every morning for the remainder of the fast. Some beneficial gut bacteria is lost during enemas, so it's very important to replenish them by eating cultured foods or taking probiotic supplements after the fast.

Enema bags can be purchased at some drugstores, natural food stores, and online. An enema bag is a rubber hot water bottle with a long tube and nozzle attached, and it can be reused many times. Follow these guidelines:

- Warm 4 cups of purified water to body temperature.
- Pour the water into the enema bag.
- Release the clamp and let the water run through the tube into a sink or tub to clear the air in the tube. Clamp the tube shut.
- Hang the enema bag on a shower rod or door knob.
- Lightly coat the nozzle at the end of the tube with coconut oil or olive oil.
- Kneel on all fours (elbows and knees) and insert the nozzle into your anus.
- Release the clamp and let the water flow into the colon; breathe and relax.
- Clamp the tube to stop the water flow when you feel full. Wait, relax, and continue.
- When the bag is empty, clamp the tube and remove the nozzle from your anus.
- To distribute the water throughout the colon, lie on your back and massage your abdomen, starting on the lower left side and moving left to right across the abdomen to just below the ribs, and then returning down the right side. Alternatively, lie on your left side to start and then turn on your back, raising your hips, and then lie on your right side. Try to retain the enema from 5 to 12 minutes.
- Sit on the toilet and empty the bowels completely. This may take a few minutes.

Hot-and-Cold Water Therapy

You can stimulate lymphatic and blood circulation when showering by alternating hot and cold water after you've completed your regular shower routine. Use hot water for 1 to 2 minutes, then follow with cold water for 30 seconds, directing the cold water to all areas of your body. Repeat the sequence three times, finishing with cold water. This therapy will close your pores, bring blood to the surface, increase circulation, tighten the skin, and leave you feeling invigorated.

Nasal and Sinus Rinse

The yogic practice of using a neti pot can be included in your morning regimen to irrigate and clear the sinuses, which indirectly helps to clear the lungs. This practice is excellent for people with allergies, mucus buildup in the lungs and sinuses, or postnasal drip. It's also a useful cleansing method for people who live in cities and regularly breathe in polluted air.

The neti pot looks like a small teapot and can be found at most natural food stores and online. To use a neti pot, fill it with a saline solution and pour the solution into one nostril, tilting your head so the water flows through the sinuses and comes out the other nostril. Follow this general procedure:

- Put 8 ounces of purified water into a small saucepan and warm it to body temperature. Stir in ¼ teaspoon of fine sea salt or ½ teaspoon of coarse salt until it dissolves. The solution should taste about as salty as tears.
- Stand in front of the sink and pour half of the solution into the neti pot.
- Bend over the sink and breathe with your mouth open. Put the neti pot's spout into your right nostril. Gently bend your head forward and turn it to the left so that the left nostril is lower than the right nostril.
- Hold your head still and pour the solution into your right nostril by tilting the neti pot upward. Continue to keep your head still as the solution pours out of your left nostril or mouth; either is fine. The course of the solution will be determined by the position of your head. Continue to pour the solution into your right nostril, making sure the exiting fluid goes into the sink.
- When finished with the right side, gently blow your nose.
- Fill the neti pot with the remaining solution and repeat the procedure on the left side, finishing once again by gently blowing your nose.

Oil Pulling

Oil pulling is another practice taken from the Ayurvedic tradition. It has been praised for having endless benefits, including improving the health of the teeth, gums, and mouth. This practice simply involves swishing one tablespoon of oil in your mouth for twenty minutes in the morning. The oil draws toxins out of the mouth and also from the blood as it circulates through, which assists in the healing and detoxification of the whole body. For the best results, oil pulling can be done every morning or several times a week. Follow these guidelines:

- After you've brushed your teeth and scraped your tongue in the morning, put 1 tablespoon of cold-pressed sesame oil or coconut oil into your mouth.

- Swish the oil around in your mouth and through your teeth without swallowing it. The oil will start to get watery as your saliva mixes with it.

- Continue to swish the oil around for twenty minutes. During this time, you can do household chores, prepare food, or even take a shower. You should feel relaxed and comfortable.

- The process is complete when the oil is thin and milky.

- Spit out the oil and rinse out your mouth with water. It's preferable to spit the oil into the earth outside or into a paper towel which you can then throw into the garbage or compost. The oil could clog the pipes in your home over time.

Tongue Scraping

While you sleep at night, your body is busy clearing out toxins. Some of these toxins are deposited on your tongue. During a juice fast, your tongue might develop a thick coating or possibly taste strange when you wake up. By gently scraping this coating off first thing in the morning, you avoid reabsorbing toxins and help your breath smell better.

In Ayurveda, the sister science of yoga, tongue scraping is recommended for the health of the teeth, gums, sinuses, and digestive system. When the tongue is clean, the taste buds function optimally and are able to communicate more clearly with the rest of the body. For example, you'll get digestive secretions when you need them, and you'll also get the message that your stomach is full earlier.

A tongue scraper is generally U-shaped and can be purchased at most drugstores or natural food stores. Using a tongue scraper is more effective than brushing your tongue with your toothbrush, which tends to stir up bacteria and plaque but not remove them from your mouth. Choose a metal tongue scraper over a plastic version. Here's how to use it:

- Brush your teeth.

- Hold an end of the tongue scraper with each hand and position the rounded middle section as far back on your tongue as possible. This may cause a gag reflex, but this will decrease over time.

- Scrape forward several times, rinsing the white film off the scraper between each scraping. Be gentle but firm as you scrape, and reach as far back on the tongue as possible with each scrape.

- Rinse your mouth with water.

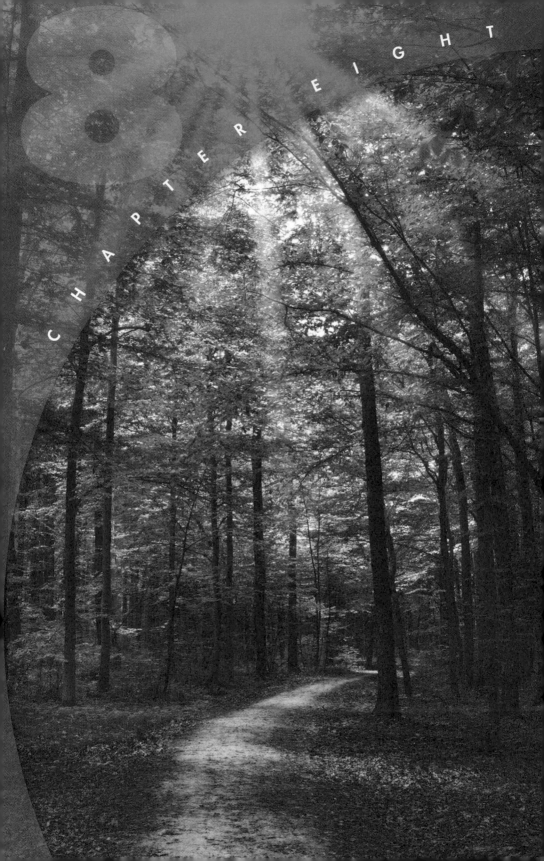

CHAPTER EIGHT

The Everyday Deep-Healing Diet

Your Mother is in you, and you in her. She bore you:
she gives you life. It was she who gave you your body,
and to her shall you one day give it back. Happy are you
when you come to know her and her kingdom; if you receive
your Mother's angels and if you do her laws. I tell you truly,
he who does these things shall never see disease. For the power
of our Mother is above all.

THE ESSENE GOSPEL OF PEACE, TRANSLATED
BY EDMOND BORDEAUX SZEKELY

A health-supportive diet is composed of real food, made by nature and unprocessed. For the times that you're not fasting, I recommend a whole-foods, plant-based diet. Yet even in the world of whole-foods nutrition there is controversy: cooked or raw food, fruit or no fruit, grains or no grains, and so on. For every expert who says that a particular food is "bad" for you, there's one who says it's "good" for you.

Try not to allow these external messages to influence you. I've consistently urged you to listen to yourself and trust your instincts during the process of deep healing. The same is true when it comes to a deep-healing diet. Let your intuition and wisdom guide you. We'll explore the physical, mental, emotional, and spiritual aspects of diet later in this chapter in the section called "Making Peace with Food" (see page 80).

First I'd like to offer a flexible formula for getting all the healthful nutrition you need from your food. As always, I urge you to listen to your body and, if necessary, consult a holistic nutritionist or other practitioner to help you refine your healing diet.

Food Sensitivities

You may be sensitive to some foods, including whole foods such as citrus fruits, corn, dairy products, eggs, glutenous grains, nuts, peanuts, pork, red meat, or soy. Sensitivities may occur because these foods have been sprayed with pesticides, have other chemical residues, have been genetically modified, or are rancid. Continuing to consume foods that you are sensitive to can contribute to physical discomforts, such as bloating, fatigue, frequent illness, inflammation, skin issues, sleep disturbances, and weight gain. Once your body has healed sufficiently, you may be able to add limited amounts of these foods back into your diet, providing you choose high-quality versions or prepare them in ways that make them easier to digest. For example, buy organic foods, including ripe citrus fruits and corn, and soak raw nuts and sprout whole grains.

DEEP-HEALING STAPLES

I n chapter 7, I introduced freshly pressed juice, mineral broths, and tea infusions. In this chapter, I'll discuss green smoothies, the Hearty Salad Meal, and the Heaven on Earth Bowl. Recipes for all of these are provided in the recipe section (pages 87 to 119).

Every day, include three or more of the following selections:

- Freshly pressed juice
- Green smoothie
- Hearty Salad Meal
- Heaven on Earth Bowl
- Mineral broth
- Tea infusion

If you include most of the above selections and snack on fresh fruit and raw vegetables, you'll have a full day's worth of healthful eating. And even if you dine out in the evening, you'll have done a lot to support your body when you drink a nourishing tea infusion or mineral broth followed by a green smoothie in the morning, have a Hearty Salad Meal at lunch, and snack on some fruit in the afternoon. You may even find something like a Heaven on Earth Bowl on the menu!

Green Smoothies

A green smoothie is a blended drink that contains fresh or frozen fruit and fresh green vegetables, including leafy greens or wild greens. A meal in a glass that you can carry with you when you're on the go, a green smoothie can be made in less than five minutes and provides an abundance of nutrients that alkalize the system.

Because the blender breaks down the hard-to-digest cellulose in leafy greens, the nutrients in green smoothies are highly absorbable and easy on the system. To make a smoothie even more nutritious, add algaes, such as chlorella, blue-green algae, or spirulina; grass juice powders, such as barley, kamut or wheat; or seeds, such as chia, flax, or hemp. Some seeds, such as flaxseeds, should be ground before using.

You can create endless combinations when making a green smoothie. Let your intuition guide you. To get started, try the Apple and Berry Smoothie (page 111) and the Chocolatey Green Shake (page 112).

Hearty Salad Meals

Make a big salad the center of at least one of your meals every day. Start by mixing the dressing, such as a basic oil-and-vinegar dressing, in the bottom of a big salad bowl. Then add ingredients that appeal to you. Start with vegetables that will hold up well in the dressing, especially if you're not planning to eat the salad right away but are packing it to take to work. Avocado, beets, cabbage, carrots, and radishes are good choices. Then add lettuce, sprouts, and nuts or seeds, along with any other vegetables you want to use. Mix just before eating.

Some hearty ingredients, such as avocado, cooked legumes or vegetables, nuts, olives, seeds, and sprouts, can turn a salad into a meal. Try the Basic Hearty Salad Meal (page 114). On days that you want something more substantial, add a soup or crackers and a dip.

Heaven on Earth Bowls

My favorite way to combine steamed vegetables, legumes, and grains is in a meal I call Heaven on Earth Bowls. I chose that name because that's how it feels when I eat them! Also, I deeply believe that the more we eat this way, the closer we get to creating heaven on earth. This one-bowl meal incorporates many of the superfoods that make up a truly health-supportive plant-based diet.

I particularly like that this meal combines cooked and raw foods. Most people don't have the physical or emotional capacity to adopt a completely raw diet and stay balanced. Properly prepared cooked foods add warmth, satisfaction, and nutrition to our daily food choices. Gently steaming or boiling vegetables makes them more digestible and warming. Well-prepared legumes help us to stay centered and grounded, and their protein content is deeply satisfying. In addition, lentils and mung beans can be sprouted and added raw to your meals. Whole unbroken grains, such as brown rice, millet, and quinoa, satisfy your carbohydrate needs in a healthy way and complement legumes nicely. Vegetables, legumes, and whole grains contain a vast array of fatty acids, fiber, minerals, phytonutrients, and protein.

A Heaven on Earth Bowl features layers of ingredients, generally starting with a base of gluten-free grains or cooked yams or squash followed by steamed or raw vegetables and delicious raw toppings. Because you can use an endless combination of ingredients, no two Heaven on Earth Bowls are the same. Be creative in assembling them, using what you have on hand and local produce that's in season. A bonus is that this meal can be made quickly using very few pans and dishes, so clean-up is a breeze.

As a nutritionist, I love this meal for a number of reasons. The ingredients are both nourishing and cleansing, and they're also satisfying yet easy to digest. The grains are wholesome and the vegetables are abundant, which is ideal because vegetables should make up at least half of the diet. In addition, the toppings are raw, so they're fresh and alive. Low in acid-forming foods, the Heaven on Earth Bowl helps to promote alkalinity. This meal is also low in fat because it's prepared with no cooked oils or frying; the addition of cold-pressed oils as a topping is optional.

Heaven on Earth Bowl Layers

I've included a Basic Heaven on Earth Bowl recipe on page 116, but the following suggestions for the various layers can help you create your own. I often steam the vegetables directly on top of the cooking grains in a tiered vegetable steamer. This method saves energy, but mostly I like that the juices from the vegetables flavor the grains and no nutrients are lost. I layer the cooked ingredients in large bowls made by a local potter and eat with wooden utensils. And I like to put the raw toppings on the table in individual bowls and let people garnish their own meals.

BASE OPTIONS
- Basmati rice, black rice, brown rice (short- or long-grain), jasmine rice, red rice, or wild rice
- Brown rice noodles (available in a variety of shapes)
- Millet
- Orange vegetables, such as winter squash or sweet potatoes
- Quinoa (white, black, red, or a combination)
- Soba noodles made from 100 percent buckwheat

DEEP HEALING
Diet and Lifestyle Lead to Longevity

Researchers who study the longest-lived populations have found that they share many common behaviors. The primary commonality is that they eat a low-calorie, plant-based diet made up of a variety of whole foods. They also tend to grow their own foods and include all food groups, such as leafy greens and root vegetables, fruits, grains, legumes, nuts and seeds, and the occasional animal-based food. In addition, in regions where locals routinely live into their nineties and even beyond, people are physically active every day—they walk to the market, tend the garden, and visit friends on foot. They also have a sense of purpose, feel deeply supported by their communities, and have faith in something greater than themselves. For further reading on longevity, I suggest the books *Healthy at 100* by John Robbins and *The Blue Zones* by Dan Buettner.

VEGETABLE OPTIONS

- One or more green leafy vegetables, such as bok choy, collard greens, kale, rapini, spinach, or Swiss chard (remove stems from collard greens and kale)
- One or more orange vegetables, such as carrot, sweet potato, or winter squash (acorn, butternut, or delicata)
- One pungent vegetable (optional), such as leek, onion, or shallot
- One member of the brassica family (optional), such as broccoli, Brussels sprouts, cabbage, or cauliflower
- Other vegetables (optional), such as a bell pepper or zucchini

TOPPING OPTIONS

- Cold-pressed oil, such as flax, hemp, olive, pumpkin, or sesame
- Fermented vegetables, such as kimchi or sauerkraut
- Fresh herbs, such as basil, chives, cilantro, parsley, or thyme
- Nuts (chopped), such as almonds, brazil nuts, or cashews
- Nutritional yeast
- Sea salt (celtic, Himalayan, or other high-quality salt), salt-free seasonings, or sea salt and herb combinations
- Sea vegetables, such as dulse flakes or crumbled nori
- Seeds, such as hemp, pumpkin, or sunflower
- Sprouts, such as alfalfa, broccoli, clover, lentil, mung bean, radish, or sunflower
- Tamari, reduced-sodium

MAKING PEACE WITH FOOD

ost people are aware that food has a profound effect on health and have tried numerous dietary approaches. And yet, most people I meet are not happy about the way they eat and feel, and many are confused about what they should be eating.

One of the key steps toward making peace with food is to realize that eating behaviors are multifaceted. Food choices are a response to physical, mental, emotional, and spiritual factors. To make peace with food, you must address all of these aspects.

Physical: Give Your Body What It Needs

Every body needs nutrients and calories from food in order for the cells and systems to function well. However, many of us are nutrient starved even though we take in plenty of calories. The most nutrient-dense foods are whole, fresh, organic, and properly prepared. It's no wonder we feel profoundly dissatisfied when we rely on poor-quality, processed foods that are stripped of nutrients.

Your physical body is made up of energy, and the food you eat has a tremendous influence on your energy body. Many foods in the modern diet decrease the body's frequency level and make us vulnerable to disease. Such foods are canned, genetically modified, processed, and sprayed with chemicals. In addition, any foods that are produced with an element of human, animal, or planetary suffering can decrease the body's frequency level.

Our task is to pay attention to how our bodies respond to food. This awareness will enable us to refine our choices on an ongoing basis. We can make adjustments based on a number of factors. One may simply be the weather. We must also pay attention to our health conditions and the physical demands of the moment. And beyond observing physical needs, we need to evaluate where we're at emotionally, energetically, and spiritually.

Mental: Question Your Food Beliefs

Much of the confusion we experience regarding food comes from the unending stream of conflicting nutritional information we see in advertisements, books, Internet blogs, and magazine and newspaper articles. If you rely too heavily on your conditioned and educated mind and its need for proof and scientific facts, you'll forever be pulled in various dietary directions. The best way to avoid confusion is to involve intuition in your lifestyle decisions. Intuition is intelligence outside of thought that arises from the place where body and soul meet, and it's the most valuable tool you have. Deep healing is impossible without honoring and nurturing intuition.

When You Eat

Your body is constantly providing information regarding the suitability of your food selections. Slow down and pay attention! Eat without distractions in a relaxed environment, and bring as much awareness as possible to your body.

Before you eat, ask yourself the following questions:

- Am I hungry?
- What do I need?
- What food would feel satisfying right now?
- Do I feel like eating something cold or warm, dense or light, salty or sweet?

While you're eating, ask yourself the following questions:

- How does the food look?
- Can I appreciate the unique beauty of whole foods, including the colors, intricate details, and shapes?
- How does the food smell?
- How does the food taste?
- Does the taste change as I chew?
- Am I rushing or enjoying?

After you eat, ask yourself the following questions:

- Do I feel satisfied?
- Does my body feel happy?
- Do I need more food or something else?
- Do I feel tired or uncomfortable?

Notice all of these things with openness and curiosity. If judgment and uncomfortable emotions come up, then bring those into your kind awareness too. Allow pleasure, enjoyment, and appreciation into your experience too. Notice where you feel the emotions in your body. Can you allow them to be as they are? If it's difficult to accept these feelings with gentleness, try to make peace with the fact that you can't accept them at this time.

To access intuition, let go of everything you think you know about food. When you have a willingness to listen to your body, you'll discover the deep-healing diet that works for you. You'll know what's right because some choices will make you feel good while others will give you uncomfortable symptoms. Be kind and patient with yourself. Let go of perfectionism and bring awareness and sincerity to the process. Stay open. With this attitude, you'll find your food choices shifting on their own.

When you're at peace and ready to connect with your intuition, the resources you need will naturally come to you. At just the right time, you'll be led to sincere practitioners, including authors and teachers, who will provide the input you need. They'll confirm what you have already intuited, answer your questions, and offer a gentle nudge into a whole new world of possibilities. Their teachings can shorten your learning curve and give you practical skills that make it easier to embrace a holistic lifestyle. When you approach healing from a place of inner peace, the path to healing will be presented to you simply and elegantly, and you'll have no need to rush frantically from one expert or one diet to the next.

Emotional: Emotions Drive Food Choices

The root causes of emotional eating are sometimes innocent and sometimes not. When we're young, parents and other caregivers offer us rich, starchy, and sweet foods to soothe us. As we grow, we're targeted by big businesses that sell convenience foods and fast foods, and these businesses cash in on food addictions that start early and may last for life. And as adults, even when we're relatively conscientious eaters, we can find ourselves overeating or constantly snacking as we look for the temporary satisfaction and distraction that food brings us.

When difficult emotions surface in the course of our days, we have a choice. We can explore the emotion to find out what it's trying to teach us, or we can avoid or suppress it with busyness; eating; drinking or drug use; excessive spending; overworking; or tuning out of the real world and into cell phones, computers, and television. Until we're deeply committed to our spiritual unfolding and deep healing, many of us will choose to avoid emotions. And eating is one of the most socially acceptable ways to do this. In fact, we all do it together!

Emotional detoxification occurs when we make more wholesome food choices. Let me explain how this works in terms of energy frequencies. When we decide to adopt a higher-vibration diet composed of whole, plant-based foods, lower-vibration energy pockets that contain suppressed emotions start to dissolve. This, of course, is positive in the long term, but in the short term we can experience uncomfortable emotions during the detoxification process. Unless we have developed the tools to deal with these emotions, we typically begin to crave lower-vibration foods again. The frustrating cycle that so many people find themselves in perpetuates itself.

I find that many people mentally establish dietary standards that they're not emotionally capable of maintaining. They grab on to an ideal and try to enforce it without considering the energetic shifts they're triggering. The only solution is to slow down and listen to the body, while making emotional awareness an ongoing commitment.

Surrounding Energies

As you increase the amount of whole, plant-based, and living foods in your diet and incorporate regular deep-healing juice fasts, your personal energy frequency levels begin to rise and you can become much more sensitive to lower-frequency and dissonant energies. Know that the increased sensitivity you feel, along with your increased interest in spirituality and simpler living, is very real indeed. Here are some of the things you might be more sensitive to:

- bars, malls, restaurants, and other places where groups of people gather, often to satisfy their addictions
- certain sections of the grocery store, especially where dairy products, eggs, seafood, and meat are displayed
- electromagnetic energy from devices such as cell phones, computers, and televisions
- large city centers
- noise
- other people's energy
- radio, television, and other media

As always, the solution is to bring your awareness to your new aversions. As you make dietary changes, you may also need to minimize your exposure to dissonant frequencies when you can, strengthen your energy field with spiritual practices, and create opportunities for yourself to recharge on an ongoing basis.

The best deep-healing food choices come from a place of inspiration and peace. When we connect to a desire to make peace with food, what we're really saying is that we're tired of the negative emotions associated with our food choices. We sense that it's possible to create a joyful and easy relationship with food that supports both the body and soul.

So many of us have tied up our precious life force battling with food. The truth is there is no battle and there has never been one. We fight food or habits that we've been led to believe are bad. Food, any type of food, is neither good nor bad in and of itself. The fact is, certain foods make us feel more or less alive physically and spiritually. If you want to be physically and spiritually vital, it's up to you to commit to this goal with your whole being. This commitment requires paying attention to your body's feedback. Only you know what brings you clarity, contentment, energy, lightness, and satisfaction. And these are only some of the uplifting and positive qualities you can enjoy on an ongoing basis when you find the most healing foods for you.

Spiritual: Connect to Peace

Don't make food less important than it is and don't make food more important than it is. Instead, try to make peace with food. This happens in four stages:

STAGE ONE. In the first stage, people give little or no thought to what they eat. They're simply eating and seemingly enjoying what feels good in the moment, what they've been raised on, and what advertisers encourage them to put into their bodies. These people are making food less important than it is, and they're not doing what is necessary to take even basic care of the human body.

STAGE TWO. When people start to feel bad physically, they may begin to question their food choices. They start educating themselves and setting new dietary standards. They tend to get rigid about their food choices and label foods as "good" or "bad." They may begin to feel better physically but aren't as joyful as they should be. Their tendency is to swing back and forth between often extreme dietary approaches, fall off the wagon, feel bad, convince themselves they can do better with willpower, and so on. This stage is where most people who have a dawning awareness about food get stuck. They make food more important than it is, overriding emotional and spiritual factors.

STEP THREE. This stage requires the biggest leap. In order to find joy and ease in eating, people realize they must begin to trust their bodies and souls to guide them to the best choices. Learning to listen to the body, and connect to the soul, requires them to clear emotional energies that have been laid down over the course of a lifetime. These energies block intuition. This stage is challenging and requires people to evolve spiritually and successfully manage the process of emotional detoxification. When we make spiritual evolution our greatest priority, we will access the strength and stamina to do this work. Until then, we continue to avoid facing difficult emotions and live on the surface of life lost in our distractions and addictions.

STAGE FOUR. People who have done the emotional work and achieved spiritual awareness are able to make food choices that reflect their ease and joy. They naturally crave high-quality foods and love the energy, inspiration, and lightness they feel. These and other positive feelings come from eating in a way that nurtures both the body and the soul.

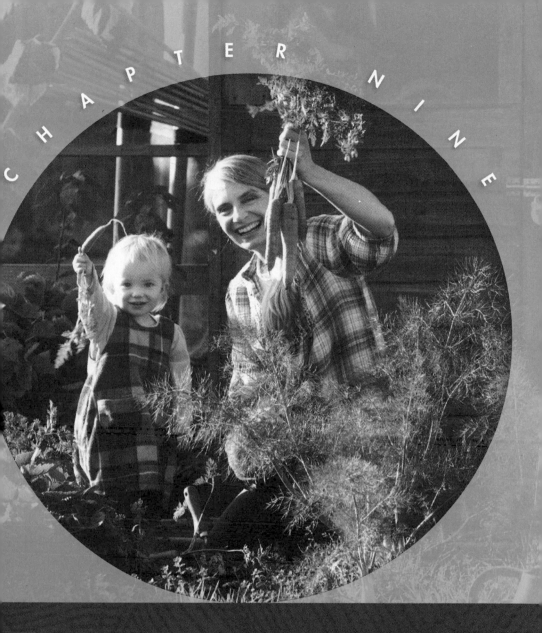

Recipes

"The doctor of the future will no longer treat the human frame with drugs,
but rather will cure and prevent disease with nutrition."

THOMAS EDISON

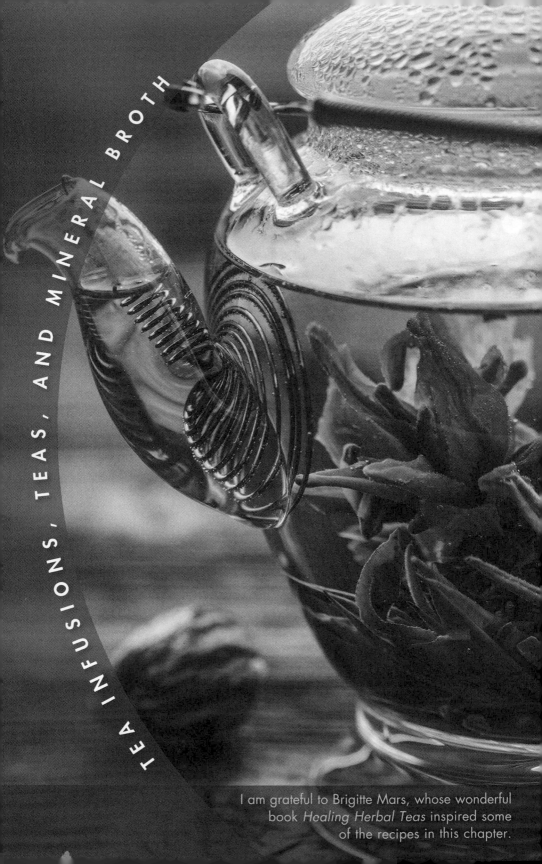

TEA INFUSIONS, TEAS, AND MINERAL BROTH

I am grateful to Brigitte Mars, whose wonderful book *Healing Herbal Teas* inspired some of the recipes in this chapter.

NOURISHING *Tea Infusion*

This all-purpose tea deeply nourishes the bones, organs, and tissues. It's ideal for all members of the family, including children and pets. To read about the many benefits of nettle leaves, oat straw, raspberry leaves, and red clover blossoms, see page 58.

1 CUP DRIED **nettle** LEAVES

1 CUP DRIED **raspberry** LEAVES

1 CUP DRIED **red clover** BLOSSOMS

½ CUP DRIED **alfalfa** LEAVES

½ CUP DRIED **oat straw**

¼ CUP DRIED **peppermint** LEAVES (optional)

4 CUPS **water**, BOILED AND SETTLED

1 Combine all the herbs in a glass container. Cover tightly and store in a cool, dark place until ready to use.

2 To make an infusion, put ½ to ¾ cup of the herb mixture in a 1-quart jar.

3 Pour the water over the herb mixtre.

4 Let the herbs steep in the water for 1 hour.

5 Pour through a strainer into a clean jar or teapot.

6 Drink immediately, while warm. Store leftover tea infusion in a sealed glass jar in the refrigerator. It will keep for 3 days. If desired, warm the leftover tea infusion before drinking.

FASTING *Tea Infusion*

A useful addition to the seven-day deep-healing juice fast, this tea is the perfect choice to cleanse the body and curb the appetite.

1 CUP **dandelion** ROOT

1 CUP **fennel** SEEDS

1 CUP DRIED **nettle** LEAVES

1 CUP DRIED **peppermint** LEAVES

1 CUP DRIED **red clover** LEAVES

1 Combine all the herbs in a glass container. Cover tightly and store in a cool, dark place until ready to use.

2 To make an infusion, put ½ to ¾ cup of the herb mixture in a 1-quart jar.

3 Pour the water over the herb mixture.

4 Let the herbs steep in the water for 1 hour.

5 Pour through a strainer into a clean jar or teapot.

6 Drink immediately, while warm.

note: Store leftover tea infusion in a sealed glass jar in the refrigerator. It will keep for 3 days. If desired, warm the leftover tea infusion before drinking.

RELAXING *Tea Infusion*

MAKES 4 CUPS

Rest and peace are both essential for deep healing. This tea infusion is an excellent choice when you need something to help you to sleep. It can also be calming during stressful times.

2 CUPS DRIED **chamomile** FLOWERS

2 CUPS DRIED **oat straw**

1 CUP DRIED **lemon balm** LEAVES

1 CUP DRIED **catnip** LEAVES

1 Combine all the herbs in a glass container. Cover tightly and store in a cool, dark place until ready to use.

2 To make an infusion, put ½ to ¾ cup of the herb mixture in a 1-quart jar.

3 Pour the water over the herb mixture.

4 Let the herbs steep in the water for 1 hour.

5 Pour through a strainer into a clean jar or teapot.

6 Drink immediately, while warm.

note: Store leftover tea infusion in a sealed glass jar in the refrigerator. It will keep for 3 days. If desired, warm the leftover tea infusion before drinking.

CALMING DIGESTIVE *Tea Infusion*

MAKES 4 CUPS

Look no further when you need something to settle and soothe your digestive system.

2 CUPS DRIED **chamomile** FLOWERS

2 CUPS **marshmallow** ROOT

1 CUP **fennel** SEEDS

1 CUP DRIED **peppermint** LEAVES

4 THIN SLICES FRESH **ginger**

1 Combine the chamomile flowers, marshmallow root, fennel seeds, and peppermint leaves in a glass container. Cover tightly and store in a cool, dark place until ready to use.

2 To make an infusion, put ½ to ¾ cup of the herbs and the ginger in a 1-quart jar.

3 Pour the water over the herbs and ginger.

4 Let the mixture steep in the water for 1 hour.

5 Pour through a strainer into a clean jar or teapot.

6 Drink immediately, while warm. Store leftover tea infusion in a sealed glass jar in the refrigerator. It will keep for 3 days. If desired, warm the leftover tea infusion before drinking.

WOMEN'S HEALTH *Tea Infusion*

MAKES 4 CUPS

Formulated especially for females, this cleansing tea infusion is nourishing and calming.

2 CUPS DRIED **nettle** LEAVES

2 CUPS DRIED **raspberry** LEAVES

1 CUP DRIED **chamomile** FLOWERS

1 CUP **dandelion** ROOT

1 CUP DRIED **rosemary** LEAVES

½ CUP **licorice** ROOT

4 THIN SLICES FRESH **ginger**

1 Combine the nettle leaves, raspberry leaves, chamomile flowers, dandelion root, rosemary leaves, and licorice root in a glass container. Cover tightly and store in a cool, dark place until ready to use.

2 To make an infusion, put ½ to ¾ cup of the herbs and the ginger in a 1-quart jar.

3 Pour the water over the herbs and ginger.

4 Let the herbs steep in the water for 1 hour.

5 Pour through a strainer into a clean jar or teapot.

6 Drink immediately, while warm. Store leftover tea infusion in a sealed glass jar in the refrigerator. It will keep for 3 days. If desired, warm the leftover tea infusion before drinking.

MEN'S HEALTH *Tea Infusion*

MAKES 4 CUPS

Especially for men, this tea infusion features herbs that benefit the heart and prostate.

1 CUP DRIED **hawthorn** BERRIES

1 CUP DRIED **nettle** LEAVES

1 CUP DRIED **oat straw**

½ CUP **cinnamon** BARK

½ CUP **fenugreek** SEEDS

4 THIN SLICES FRESH **ginger**

1 Combine the hawthorn berries, nettle leaves, oat straw, cinnamon bark, and fenugreek seeds in a glass container. Cover tightly and store in a cool, dark place until ready to use.

2 To make an infusion, put ½ to ¾ cup of the herbs and the ginger in a 1-quart jar.

3 Pour the water over the herb mixture.

4 Let the herbs steep in the water for 1 hour.

5 Pour through a strainer into a clean jar or teapot.

6 Drink immediately, while warm. Store leftover tea infusion in a sealed glass jar in the refrigerator. It will keep for 3 days. If desired, warm the leftover tea infusion before drinking.

GINGER AND LEMON *Tea*

This easy-to-make tea has warming properties, soothes the digestive system, relieves cold symptoms, and helps settle coughs.

10 THIN SLICES FRESH **ginger**

4 CUPS **water**

JUICE OF 1 **lemon**

maple syrup

1 Put the ginger and water in a small saucepan over medium heat.

2 Simmer for 20 to 30 minutes, or longer if you prefer a stronger tea.

3 Stir in the lemon juice and maple syrup to taste.

4 Serve hot.

CHAGA *Tea*

MAKES 6 CUPS

Chaga is a hard black mushroom that grows primarily on birch trees and is used to make a rich, robust, and very pleasant hot tea. Chaga tea has been used medicinally mostly in Russia but has recently become popular in North America among health enthusiasts. With high amounts of minerals and

⅓ CUP DRIED **chaga** CHUNKS

6 CUPS **water**

1 Put the chaga and water in a medium saucepan over medium heat.

2 Simmer for 30 minutes.

3 Strain.

4 Drink immediately, while warm. Store leftover Chaga Tea in a sealed glass jar in the refrigerator. It will keep for 3 days. Warm the leftover tea before drinking.

antioxidants, the tea is used as a remedy and preventive for cancer, but it also has antibacterial, antifungal, and antiviral properties. You can purchase dried chaga chunks at a natural food store; the chunks are costly but can be used three or four times.

notes

- The chaga chunks can be reused three or four times. One way to reuse the chunks is to add more water each time you take some tea from the saucepan and let the tea simmer for about another 15 minutes. Keep adding water until the tea becomes pale.

- The second option is to serve all the tea, add another 6 cups of water to the saucepan with the chaga chunks, and simmer for 30 minutes. You can do this three or four times, until the tea becomes pale.

- A third option is handy when you don't need a lot of tea all at once. Put the used, moist chaga chunks in a small container and store them in the freezer until you're ready to make more tea. The chunks can be reused and refrozen three or four times.

MINERAL *Broth*

Making mineral broth is an easy and economical way to use up vegetables that are past their prime and vegetable parts that you would otherwise compost (see note). Adding sea vegetables to the broth increases the nutritional value. Enjoy mineral broth on its own or use it as a rich base for soups or as the cooking liquid for grains. No two mineral broths are the same, but this basic recipe can get you started.

2 **carrots**, COARSELY CHOPPED

2 **potatoes**, COARSELY CHOPPED

1 **beet**, COARSELY CHOPPED

1 **celery root**, COARSELY CHOPPED (optional)

1 **onion**, COARSELY CHOPPED

1 **sweet potato**, COARSELY CHOPPED (optional)

2 CUPS COARSELY CHOPPED **kale** LEAVES, LIGHTLY PACKED, OR KALE STEMS

1 CUP COARSELY CHOPPED **cabbage** OR CABBAGE CORE

1 CUP COARSELY CHOPPED DARK **leek greens**

½ CUP CHOPPED FRESH **parsley**, LIGHTLY PACKED

1 SHEET **nori**, TORN

1 STRIP **kombu**

1 TABLESPOON **dulse flakes**

1 TABLESPOON CHOPPED FRESH **thyme** OR **oregano**

2 **bay leaves**

1 Put all the ingredients in a large soup pot and add enough water to cover the vegetables by 2 inches.

2 Bring to a boil over high heat. Decrease the heat to medium-low, cover, and simmer for 3 hours. The vegetables will be very soft and discolored.

3 Set a colander over a large bowl and strain the broth. Then pour the strained broth through a fine-mesh strainer to remove any remaining solids.

4 Stored in a sealed container, Mineral Broth will keep for 4 days in the refrigerator or 3 months in the freezer. If freezing the broth, you may want to store it in small containers so you can thaw just the amount needed for recipes.

notes

- Feel free to use any additional vegetables you have on hand in this broth. If you're making the broth as a base for a particular soup recipe, consider the overall flavor that you want the soup to have. When making broth for certain soups, it's best to avoid strong-tasting vegetables, such as broccoli, cabbage, cauliflower, and garlic.

- Here's a handy method for collecting vegetable trimmings for broth: At the beginning of the week, put an empty container in refrigerator and put trimmings in it after preparing meals. For example, save leftover asparagus ends; broccoli, cauliflower, collard green, kale, and mushroom stems; cabbage cores; carrot and celery leaves; corn silk; and dark leek greens. By the end of the week, you will have ample trimmings to add to the broth.

- If you have liquid left over from cooking beans, you can add that to the broth too.

- For more information on mineral broths, see page 56.

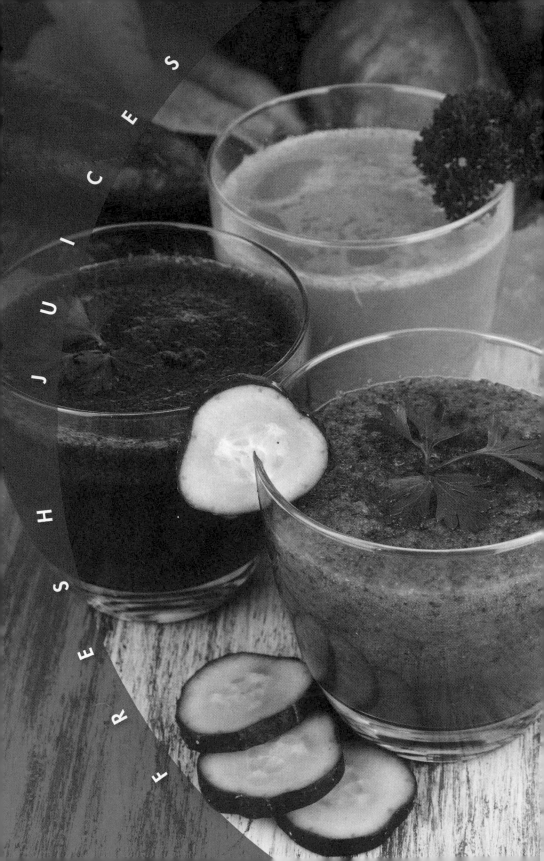

CELERY, LETTUCE, AND CUCUMBER *Juice*

This alkalizing green juice tastes mild and is excellent for the complexion and nervous system.

1 **lemon**

6 STALKS **celery**, LEAVES REMOVED

6 LEAVES **romaine lettuce**

1 **cucumber**, PEELED

1 Peel the lemon with a serrated knife, leaving some of the white pith. Cut into chunks and remove the seeds.

2 Cut the celery, lettuce, and cucumber into chunks in sizes appropriate for the juicer.

3 Run all the ingredients through the juicer, alternating the softer ingredients (the lemon and cucumber) with the denser ingredients (the celery and lettuce), and finishing with celery. This technique will help keep the juicer's blades and screens clean.

4 If desired, pour the juice through a fine-mesh strainer to remove all the pulp.

5 Serve immediately.

GAZPACHO *Juice*

This is the perfect juice to make in the summertime when tomatoes, cucumbers, and peppers are abundant and fresh.

3 STALKS **celery**, LEAVES REMOVED

1 LARGE **tomato**

1 MEDIUM **field cucumber**, PEELED

½ **red bell pepper**

1 SMALL CLOVE **garlic**

2 CUPS FRESH **spinach**, LIGHTLY PACKED

1 CUP **sunflower greens**, LIGHTLY PACKED (optional)

½ CUP FRESH **cilantro**, LIGHTLY PACKED

Salt (optional)

1 Cut the celery, tomato, cucumber, and bell pepper into chunks in sizes appropriate for the juicer.

2 Run all the vegetables through the juicer, alternating the softer vegetables, (the cucumber and tomato) with the denser vegetables (the celery and leafy greens), and finishing with celery. This technique will help keep the juicer's blades and screens clean.

3 If desired, pour the juice through a fine-mesh strainer to remove all the pulp.

4 Stir in salt to taste if desired.

5 Serve immediately.

CELERY, SPINACH, AND KALE *Juice*

MAKES 2 SERVINGS

This green juice contributes beautifully to tissue regeneration. The green apples add just a hint of sweetness.

½ **lemon**

2 **green apples**, UNPEELED AND CORED

4 STALKS **celery**

4 CUPS **spinach**, LIGHTLY PACKED

3 LEAVES **kale**

½ CUP **parsley**, LIGHTLY PACKED

1 Peel the lemon with a serrated knife, leaving some of the white pith. Cut into chunks and remove the seeds.

2 Cut the apples and celery and apple into chunks in sizes appropriate for the juicer. Depending on the juicer, you may also have to slice the spinach and kale.

3 Run all the ingredients through the juicer, alternating the softer ingredients (the lemon and apple) with the denser ingredients (the celery and leafy greens), and finishing with celery. This technique will help keep the juicer's blades and screens clean.|

4 If desired, pour the juice through a fine-mesh strainer to remove all the pulp.

5 Serve immediately.

CARROT, APPLE, AND BEET *Juice*

MAKES 2 SERVINGS

With just a hint of ginger, this deep red juice is truly heavenly. Try to consume sweet juices like this one about twenty minutes prior to or after physical activity so that you quickly burn the abundant natural sugars.

6 **carrots**, SCRUBBED

2 **green apples**, UNPEELED AND CORED

1 **beet**

½ **lemon**

½ INCH FRESH **ginger**

1 Peel the lemon with a serrated knife, leaving some of the white pith. Cut into chunks and remove the seeds.

2 Cut the carrots, apples, and beet into chunks in sizes appropriate for the juicer.

3 Run the ingredients through the juicer, alternating the softer ingredients the apples and lemon) with the denser ingredients (the beet and carrots), and finishing with carrot. This technique will help keep the juicer's blades and screens clean.

4 If desired, pour the juice through a fine-mesh strainer to remove all the pulp.

5 Serve immediately.

CARROT, APPLE, AND FENNEL *Juice*

MAKES 2 SERVINGS

This juice provides a terrific way to use up the stems when you include fresh fennel bulbs in salads and other dishes.

5 **carrots**

2 **green apples**, UNPEELED AND CORED

2 **oranges**

3 OR 4 **fennel stems** WITH LEAVES

1 Cut the carrots, apples, and oranges into chunks in sizes appropriate for the juicer.

2 Run all the ingredients through the juicer, alternating the softer ingredients (the apples and oranges) with the denser ingredients (the carrots and fennel), and finishing with carrot. This technique will help keep the juicer's blades and screens clean.

3 If desired, pour the juice through a fine-mesh strainer to remove all the pulp.

4 Serve immediately.

CITRUS AND GREENS *Juice*

MAKES 2 SERVINGS

This juice is energizing and the perfect choice for mornings when you need a little extra boost to get going. The grapefruit helps to break up excess mucus and the greens are alkalizing and grounding.

1 **grapefruit**

1 **orange**

1 **green apple**, UNPEELED AND CORED

1 **romaine** LETTUCE HEART

2 STALKS **celery**

½ CUP **sunflower sprouts** (optional)

1 Peel the grapefruit and orange with a serrated knife, leaving some of the white pith. Cut into chunks and remove the seeds.

2 Cut the apple, lettuce, and celery into chunks in sizes appropriate for the juicer.

3 Run all the ingredients through the juicer, alternating the softer ingredients (the grapefruit, orange, and apple), with the denser ingredients (the romaine and celery), and finishing with celery. This technique will help keep the juicer's blades and screens clean.

4 If desired, pour the juice through a fine-mesh strainer to remove all the pulp.

5 Serve immediately.

APPLE AND GREENS *Juice*

Thanks to the apples, this juice is moderately sweet, making it a good introduction to green juices.

3 **green apples**, UNPEELED AND CORED

4 STALKS **celery**

4 LEAVES **kale**

4 LEAVES **dandelion**

½ INCH FRESH **ginger**

1 Cut the apples and celery into chunks in sizes appropriate for the juicer. Depending on the juicer, you may also have to slice the kale.

2 Run all the ingredients through the juicer, alternating the softest ingredient, the apples, with the denser leafy greens, and finishing with the celery. This technique will help keep the juicer's blades and screens clean.

3 If desired, pour the juice through a fine-mesh strainer to remove all the pulp.

4 Serve immediately.

ORANGE, PINEAPPLE, AND CELERY *Juice*

MAKES 2 SERVINGS

According to author Bernard Jensen, pineapple nourishes the heart, liver, and skin. This delicious combination is both refreshing and replenishing after physical activity.

2 **oranges**

2 CUPS **pineapple** CHUNKS

8 STALKS **celery**

1 Peel the orange with a serrated knife, leaving some of the white pith. Cut into chunks and remove the seeds.

2 Cut the celery into chunks in sizes appropriate for the juicer.

3 Run all the ingredients through the juicer, alternating the softer ingredients (the pineapple and oranges) with the denser celery, and finishing with celery. This technique will help keep the juicer's blades and screens clean.

4 If desired, pour the juice through a fine-mesh strainer to remove all the pulp.

5 Serve immediately.

FENNEL AND GRAPEFRUIT *Juice*

The grapefruit and celery in this intriguing juice are beneficial to the lungs and sinuses.

2 CUPS CHOPPED **fennel** (BULB OR STALKS)

2 **grapefruits**

3 STALKS **celery**

1 **green apple**

1 Cut the fennel, grapefruit, celery, and apple into chunks in sizes appropriate for the juicer..

2 Run all the ingredients through the juicer, alternating the softer ingredients (the grapefruit and apple) with the denser ingredients (the fennel and celery), and finishing with celery. This technique will help keep the juicer's blades and screens clean.

3 If desired, pour the juice through a fine-mesh strainer to remove all the pulp.

4 Serve immediately.

CUCUMBER, MINT, AND LIME Juice

Try this juice during the summer, when cucumbers are at their peak and fresh mint is abundant.

1 **lime**

1 **cucumber**, PEELED

2 **green apples**, UNPEELED AND CORED

2 STALKS **celery**

6 **mint** LEAVES

1 Peel the lime with a serrated knife, leaving some of the white pith. Cut into chunks and remove the seeds.

2 Cut the cucumber, apples, and celery into chunks in sizes appropriate for the juicer.

3 Run all the ingredients through the juicer, alternating the softer ingredients (the cucumber and apples) with the denser celery, and finishing with celery. This technique will help keep the juicer's blades and screens clean.

4 If desired, pour the juice through a fine-mesh strainer to remove all the pulp.

5 Serve immediately.

THAI GREEN *Juice*

MAKES 2 SERVINGS

Cilantro is one of the most potent removers of heavy metals. Enjoy it in this delectable and nourishing juice.

1 **lime**

2 CUPS CHOPPED **pineapple**

2 STALKS **celery**

4 LEAVES **kale**

15 SPRIGS **cilantro**

1 Peel the lime with a serrated knife, leaving some of the white pith. Cut into chunks and remove the seeds.

2 Cut the celery into chunks in sizes appropriate for the juicer. Depending on the juicer, you may also need to slice the kale.

3 Run all the ingredients through the juicer, alternating the softer ingredient (the pineapple) with the denser ingredients (the celery and kale), and finishing with celery. This technique will help keep the juicer's blades and screens clean.

4 If desired, pour the juice through a fine-mesh strainer to remove all the pulp.

5 Serve immediately.

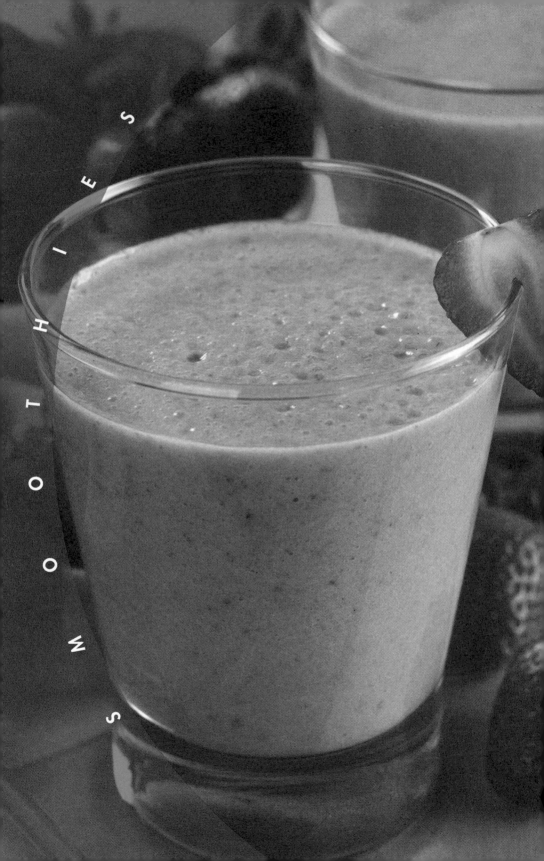

SMOOTHIES

APPLE AND BERRY *Smoothie*

MAKES 2 SERVINGS

The warming spices in this smoothie make it an ideal choice during the colder months.

2 **apples**, CORED (see notes)

2 CUPS **water**, PLUS MORE AS NEEDED (see notes)

1½ CUPS **spinach**, KALE, OR SWISS CHARD, LIGHTLY PACKED

1 CUP FRESH OR FROZEN **raspberries**, **blueberries**, OR **strawberries**

1 STALK **celery**

4 PITTED SOFT **dates**

½ INCH PEELED FRESH **ginger**

1 TABLESPOON GROUND **flaxseeds** OR **chia seeds**

1 TABLESPOON RAW **almond butter**

½ TEASPOON GROUND **cinnamon**

1 Combine all the ingredients in a blender and process until smooth. Add more water if necessary to achieve the desired consistency.

2 Serve immediately.

notes

- If desired, substitute one ripe banana for one of the apples.
- If desired, substitute part of the water with apple juice.

CHOCOLATEY GREEN *Shake*

Don't let the army-green color of this blender creation alarm you. It's delicious.

2 FRESH OR FROZEN **bananas**

1½ CUPS **water**, PLUS MORE AS NEEDED

6 PITTED SOFT **dates**

2 TABLESPOONS **hemp seeds**

1 TABLESPOON **cacao** POWDER

1 TABLESPOON **carob** POWDER

1 HEAPING TABLESPOON **almond** OR **macadamia nut butter**

¼ TEASPOON **barley grass** POWDER (see note)

¼ TEASPOON **spirulina** (see note)

PINCH **salt**

1 Combine all the ingredients in a blender and process until smooth. Add more water if necessary to achieve the desired consistency.

2 Serve immediately.

note: The amounts of the barley grass powder and spirulina can be adjusted according to your preference.

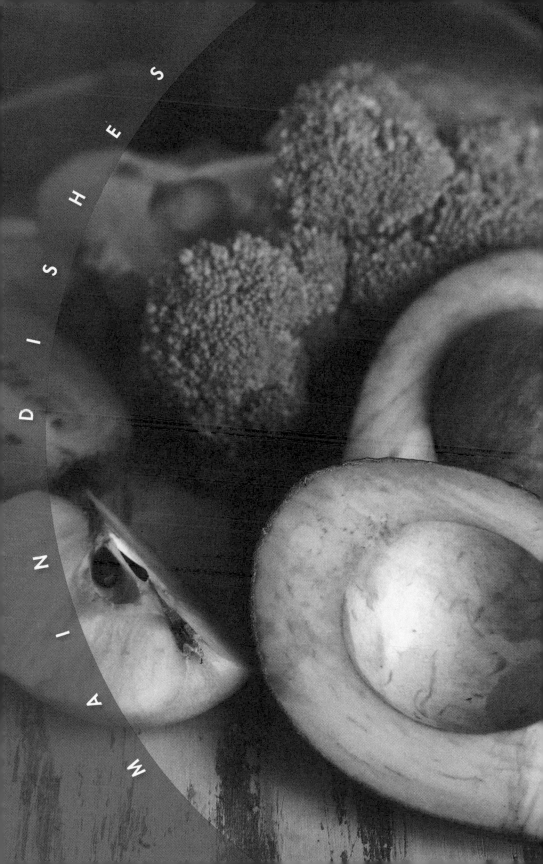

MAIN DISHES

BASIC HEARTY
SALAD *Meal*

MAKES 2 MEAL-SIZED SERVINGS OR 4 SIDE SALADS

This recipe provides just an example of the flavorful combinations you can create in a salad meal. Feel free to use your favorite fruits and vegetables, including any bits that are left over in the refrigerator. Leftover grains, legumes, or tofu are also appetizing additions.

Salad

6 CUPS CHOPPED **salad greens**, SUCH AS ROMAINE LETTUCE, GREEN OR RED LEAF LETTUCE, SPRING MIX, SPINACH, OR A COMBINATION

1 **apple**, DICED

1 **avocado**, DICED (OPTIONAL)

1 **beet**, GRATED OR COOKED AND SLICED

1 **carrot**, GRATED

1 CUP **sunflower sprouts**

1 CUP OTHER **sprouts** OR **microgreens**

½ CUP CHOPPED FRESH **cilantro** OR **parsley**, LIGHTLY PACKED

½ CUP **mung bean** OR **lentil sprouts**

½ CUP **red cabbage**, THINLY SLICED

⅓ CUP CHOPPED **walnuts** OR **pecans**

2 **green onions**, SLICED

Dressing

3 TABLESPOONS EXTRA-VIRGIN **olive oil**

1½ TABLESPOONS **cider vinegar**

1 TEASPOON **maple syrup** (optional)

½ TEASPOON **salt**

1 To make the dressing, put the oil, vinegar, optional maple syrup, and salt in a large salad bowl and whisk until well combined.

2 Add the salad ingredients and toss to combine. Serve immediately.

BASIC HEAVEN ON EARTH *Bowl*

MAKES 4 SERVINGS

Simple, flavorful, and versatile, this meal-in-a-bowl can be made with an endless variety of ingredients and toppings. The following recipe shows you how to build a Heaven on Earth Bowl layer by layer. Once you get the concept, adjust it to your preferences. Have fun!

1 CUP **quinoa**, SOAKED IN WATER FOR 4 TO 8 HOURS

1¾ CUPS **water**

3 CUPS **broccoli** FLORETS

2 **carrots**, QUARTERED LENGTHWISE AND SLICED ¼ INCH THICK

1 CUP CHOPPED FRESH **cilantro**, LIGHTLY PACKED, FOR GARNISH

1 CUP **mung bean** OR **lentil sprouts**, FOR GARNISH, PLUS OTHER SPROUTS AS DESIRED

1 CUP RAW **sauerkraut**, FOR GARNISH

⅓ CUP CHOPPED **Brazil nuts** OR **raw almonds**, FOR GARNISH

2 **green onions** OR CHIVES, THINLY SLICED, FOR GARNISH

salt OR SEASONED SALT

COLD-PRESSED **sesame oil**

1 Drain and rinse the quinoa. Transfer to a medium saucepan. Add the water and bring to a boil over high heat. Decrease the heat to medium-low, cover, and cook undisturbed for 15 to 20 minutes, until the water is absorbed and the quinoa is tender. Let stand, covered, for 5 minutes. Fluff with a fork.

2 Meanwhile, put about 1 inch of water in a medium saucepan, ideally using a vegetable steamer insert. Put the broccoli and carrots in the saucepan or insert, and bring to a boil over high heat. Decrease the heat to medium-low, cover, and cook until the vegetables are tender-crisp, about 8 minutes. Drain well. (For an alternative cooking method, see the notes.)

3 Put the cilantro, sprouts, sauerkraut, nuts, and green onions in separate small bowls on the table. Pass the salt and sesame oil at the table.

4 To serve, equally distribute the quinoa among four large soup bowls and top with the cooked vegetables. Serve immediately, letting diners garnish and season their own meals as desired.

notes:

- If you don't have time to soak the quinoa, increase the amount of water to 2 cups.
- Substitute cooked brown rice, 100 percent buckwheat soba noodles, or millet for the cooked quinoa.
- If you have a tiered vegetable steamer, cook the quinoa in the bottom and steam the vegetables one tier above the quinoa. This method will save energy. In addition, the juices from the vegetables will flavor the quinoa. Put the denser vegetables on the bottom of the steamer so they're exposed to more heat. Keep an eye on the vegetables and remove them once they are tender-crisp.
- Vary the vegetables according to what you have in the refrigerator. Always try to choose one orange and one green vegetable, since each offers unique nutritional advantages.
- For more information about Heaven on Earth Bowls, see page 77.

BASIC CULTURED *Vegetables*

Just as you can with the Hearty Salad Meal and the Heaven on Earth Bowl, you can create endless versions of cultured vegetables. Here is a basic recipe for you to start with. The red cabbage gives the finished product a pleasing pink color. Because of the fermentation process, cultured vegetables are loaded with beneficial bacteria and assist in all stages of digestion. Enjoy one or two tablespoons with any meal.

1 HEAD **cabbage**

1 CUP **red cabbage**

1 **carrot**

6 INCHES **daikon** RADISH

1 TEASPOON **sea salt**, PLUS MORE AS NEEDED

1 Wash and scrub the vegetables well. Remove the outer damaged and soft cabbage leaves and set aside.

2 Shred the cabbages and grate the carrot and radish.

3 Combine all the vegetables in a large bowl. Start by adding 1 teaspoon of the salt and add more as needed, up to 1 additional teaspoon. (See note.).

4 Massage and squeeze the vegetables with your hands until they soften and juice starts to be released. Vegetables tend to be drier in the winter, so you may need to let the vegetables sit in the salt for about 1 hour or to coax the juices out. Squeeze the vegetables once more.

5 Pack the vegetable mixture into one clean 2-liter jar or two 1-liter jars or a fermentation crock if you have one. Widemouthed jars work well. Start with about 1 cup of the mixture and pack it down with your fist, a dowel, or a potato masher, until juice rises up above the vegetables. Repeat with subsequent layers until the mixture is 2 inches from the top of the jar. There should be about

1 inch of juice above the mixture when you press down. If not, add a little saltwater to the jar.

6 Fold the reserved cabbage leaf and put it on the mixture. Top the leaf with a weight (see notes) to keep the vegetables submerged. Put the lid on the jar, letting it rest slightly askew to allow gases to escape; alternatively, cover the jar with a cloth or pillowcase secured with an elastic band to prevent dust and insects from getting in.

7 Let the mixture sit at about 70 degrees for 7 to 10 days to ferment. Put the jar on an old dish towel or in a bowl because it may sweat during the fermentation process. Fermentation takes longer in colder temperatures.

8 Start tasting the mixture after a few days to evaluate how the fermentation is progressing and determine when the taste peaks.

9 When the fermentation is complete, seal the jar tightly and store the cultured vegetables in the refrigerator to slow down the fermentation process. Unopened cultured vegetables will keep for 4 months in the refrigerator. Once they're opened, use them within 6 weeks.

notes:

- Because salt is known to inhibit the growth of unwanted bacteria, cultured vegetables and dishes such as sauerkraut have traditionally been quite salty. Today, however, some people make cultured vegetables with very little or no salt, and this works just fine. Because salt slows down fermentation in general, cultured vegetables will ferment faster when less salt is used. For example, if you were to use no salt in Cultured Vegetables, fermentation would be complete in about 5 days. I like to lightly salt the vegetables so they taste pleasingly salty.

- I suggest a couple of options for weighing down the cabbage leaf. One is to use a stone that has been boiled and sanitized. It can be fun to scout for the perfect stone when walking outdoors. Another option is to use a smaller jar that is filled with water and fits inside the opening of the larger jar. Whether using a stone, a water-filled jar, or other weight, cover the fermentation jar with a cloth secured with an elastic band to discourage pests.

Index

Recipe names and page references for sidebars appear in *italicized* typeface.

bone nourishment, tea infusion for, 87
Bowl, Basic Heaven on Earth, 116–17
brain diseases, *31*
breast cancer, *31*
breath/breathing
    asthma and, *31*
    fresh air, 7
    for lymphatic system/skin health, 44
    during meditation, *36,* 36–37
broth. *See* minerals/mineral broth(s)
brow chakra, *18, 19*
Buddhist metta practice, 1
Buettner, Dan *(The Blue Zones),* 79
B vitamins, 60

C

caffeine, 47, 54
calcium, oat straw as source for, 58
Calming Digestive Tea Infusion, 90
Campbell, Joseph, *11*
cancer
    animal-based foods and, 3
    blocked energy and, *31*
    body frequency and, 15
    castor oil and, 67
    debris contributing to, 70
    fresh juice and, *55*
    mushroom tea for, *95*
    red clover blossoms and, 58
    sunshine's effect on, 9
    wheatgrass juice and, 59
canned foods, 80
Carrot, Apple, and Beet Juice, 102
Carrot, Apple, and Fennel Juice, 103
castor oil packs, 65, 67–69
celery
    Juice, Orange, Pineapple, and, 106

Lettuce, and Cucumber Juice, 99
Spinach, and Kale Juice, 101
Chaga Tea, 94–95
chakras, 17–19, *18,* 37, 39
chemicals
    in cleaners, 45
    in foods, 42, 76, 80
    illness and, 47
    in sunscreens, 80
    as toxic, 42
    in water, 5–6, 59
chi (life force/prana), 30
children
    energy and, 12, 13, 23–24, *25, 25,* 28
    sunshine's effect on, 9
    tea infusion for, 87
Chocolatey Green Shake, 112
choices, about healing, 3–4
cilantro, to remove heavy metals/in green juice, 109
Citrus and Greens Juice, 104
cleansing. *See* detoxification (cleansing)
coffee, avoiding/effect on body, 45, 54, 57
cold symptoms, tea for, 93
colitis, *31*
collective energy(ies), *14,* 29
collective fear, 48
colon, caring for, 46
colonics/enemas, 44, 60, 65, 70–71
comfort/discomfort, during deep healing, 5
community's role in healing, 6
complexion, fresh juice for, 99
conditioning/conditioned self, 22, 28, 41
constipation, *31,* 43
cosmetics, 42, 45
coughs, tea for, 93
Cousens, Gabriel *(Spiritual Nutrition and the Rainbow Diet),* 51

creativity
    about, 6–7
    deep-healing affecting, 41
    false beliefs blocking, 23
    flow of energy and, 11
    gallstones and, *31*
    prostate disease and, *31*
    sacral chakra and, 17
    toxins and, 42
crown chakra, *18,* 19
Cucumber, Mint, and Lime Juice, 108
Cucumber Juice, Celery, Lettuce, and, 99
Cultured Vegetables, Basic, 118–19

D

dairy products
    avoiding, respiratory/urinary systems and, 45
    digestive difficulty and, 60
    disease and, 3
    energy/sensitivity and, 13–14, *83*
    food sensitivity and, 76
debris, in colon, 70
deep listening, 3, 16, 39
detoxification (cleansing). *See also* specific types of
    about, 2–3, 41
    food choices and, 43–45
    healing crisis and, 46–47
    sources of toxins, 42–43
    spiritual lessons and, 46
    tea infusion for, 88
    trust during, 47–48
    week-long cleanse, 53, 65
diabetes, 3, *31,* 48, 55
diet
    about, 75
    food sensitivities and, 76
    healing and, xiii, 2
    illness and, 30
    juice fasting and, 54, 60
    longevity and, 79
    making peace with food and, 80–84
    plant-based, 3

Acknowledgements

I would like to express my deep gratitude to my spiritual teachers Adyashanti, Sharon Landrith, Mukti, and Thomas Huebl for their role in my unfolding; Robert Warren for deepening my understanding of deep healing through our work together; Dr. Mary O'Reilly for her support and encouragement on my healing journey; the many people that I encounter in my health practice for their courage, beauty, and trust; and Jo Stepaniak, Cynthia Holzapfel, and Ellen Foreman, for their meticulous work and care in the editing and design process.

About the Author

aroline Marie Dupont, M.Sc. has been exploring, living, and teaching an integrated approach to health for over 25 years. She has a master's degree in exercise physiology, is a holistic nutritionist, yoga teacher, and energy worker, and a senior instructor at the Canadian School of Natural Nutrition. She has taught food preparation, meditation, movement and nutrition, and offers the Deep Healing Course and ClearBeing Retreats, as well as private consultations. She is the author of the bestselling book *The New Enlightened Eating*. Her website is www.carolinedupont.com.

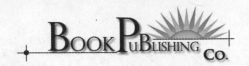

BOOK PUBLISHING CO.

books that educate, inspire, and empower

To find your favorite vegetarian and soyfood products online, visit:
healthy-eating.com

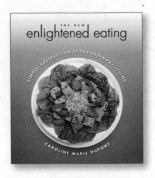

**The New
Enlightened Eating**

Caroline Marie Dupont

978-0-92047-083-1

$19.95

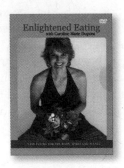

**Enlightened Eating
(DVD)**

Caroline Marie Dupont

620193000559

$19.95

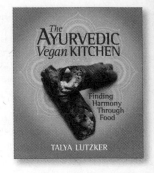

**The Ayurvedic
Vegan Kitchen**

Talya Lutzker

978-1-57067-286-6

$19.95

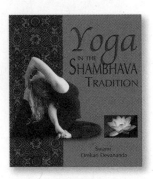

**Yoga in the
Shambhava Tradition**

Swami Omkari Devananda

978-1-57067-199-9

$29.95

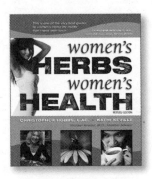

**Women's Herbs,
Women's Health**

*Christopher Hobbs, LAc,
Kathi Keville*

978-1-57067-152-4

$24.95

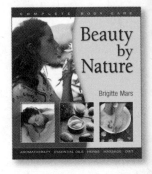

Beauty by Nature

Brigitte Mars

978-1-57067-193-7

$19.95

Purchase these health titles and cookbooks from your local bookstore or natural food store,
or you can buy them directly from:

Book Publishing Company • P.O. Box 99 • Summertown, TN 38483 • 800-695-2241

Please include $3.95 per book for shipping and handling.